A Pill for Promiscuity

Q+ Public books are a limited series of curated volumes, inspired by the seminal journal *OUT/LOOK: National Lesbian and Gay Quarterly.* *OUT/LOOK* built a bridge between academic inquiry and the broader community. Q+ Public promises to revitalize a queer public sphere to bring together activists, intellectuals, and artists to explore questions that urgently concern all LGBTQ+ communities.

Series editors: E. G. Crichton, Jeffrey Escoffier (from 2018–2022)

E. G. Crichton, *Matchmaking in the Archive: 19 Conversations with the Dead and 3 Encounters with Ghosts*
Shantel Gabrieal Buggs and Trevor Hoppe, eds., *Unsafe Words: Queering Consent in the #MeToo Era*
Andrew Spieldenner and Jeffrey Escoffier, eds., *A Pill for Promiscuity: Gay Sex in an Age of Pharmaceuticals*

A Pill for Promiscuity

Gay Sex in an Age of
Pharmaceuticals

EDITED BY ANDREW SPIELDENNER
AND JEFFREY ESCOFFIER

Rutgers University Press
New Brunswick, Camden, and Newark, New Jersey
London and Oxford, UK

Rutgers University Press is a department of Rutgers, The State University of New Jersey, one of the leading public research universities in the nation. By publishing worldwide, it furthers the University's mission of dedication to excellence in teaching, scholarship, research, and clinical care.

Library of Congress Cataloging-in-Publication Data
Names: Spieldenner, Andrew R., 1972– editor. | Escoffier, Jeffrey, editor.
Title: A pill for promiscuity : gay sex in an age of pharmaceuticals /
edited by Andrew R. Spieldenner and Jeffrey Escoffier.
Description: New Brunswick : Rutgers University Press, [2023] |
Series: Q+ public | Includes bibliographical references and index.
Identifiers: LCCN 2022013772 | ISBN 9781978824560 (hardback) |
ISBN 9781978824553 (paperback) | ISBN 9781978824577 (epub) |
ISBN 9781978824591 (pdf)
Subjects: LCSH: Gay men—Sexual behavior. | AIDS (Disease)—Prevention. |
HIV infections—Prevention. | Pre-exposure prophylaxis | BISAC: SOCIAL SCIENCE
/ LGBTQ+ Studies / Gay Studies | HEALTH & FITNESS / Sexuality Classification:
LCC HQ 76.115 .P55 2023 | DDC 306.77086/642—dc23/eng/20221005
LC record available at https://lccn.loc.gov/2022013772

A British Cataloging-in-Publication record for this book is available
from the British Library.

References to internet websites (URLs) were accurate at the time of writing.
Neither the author nor Rutgers University Press is responsible for URLs that
may have expired or changed since the manuscript was prepared.

∞ The paper used in this publication meets the requirements of the
American National Standard for Information Sciences—Permanence of Paper
for Printed Library Materials, ANSI Z39.48-1992.

rutgersuniversitypress.org

Manufactured in the United States of America

The willingness to have sex immediately, promiscuously, with people about whom one knows nothing and from whom one demands only physical contact, can be seen as a sort of Whitmanesque democracy, a desire to know and trust other men in a type of brotherhood far removed from the male bonding of rank, hierarchy, and competition that characterizes much of the outside world.
—Dennis Altman, *The Homosexualization of America*, pp. 79–80

Contents

Series Foreword

Q+ Public is a series of small thematic books in which leading scholars, artists, community leaders and activists, independent writers and thinkers engage in critical reflection on contemporary LGBTQ political, social and cultural issues.

Why Q+ Public? It invites all of the L, the G, the B, the T, the Q, and any other sexual and gender minorities. It asserts the need and existence of a Queer public space. It is also a riff on "John Q. Public" stripped of his gender, and even on Star Trek's "Q Continuum"! Q+ Public is about elevating the challenges of thinking about gender, sex, and sexuality in contemporary life.

Q+ Public is an outgrowth, after a long hibernation, of *OUT/LOOK Lesbian and Gay Quarterly*, a pioneering political and cultural journal that sparked intense national debate during the time it was published in San Francisco, 1988 to 1992. *OUT/LOOK*, in turn, spawned the *OutWrite* conferences that started in San Francisco in 1990 and 1991, then moved to Boston for a number of years.

We plan to revive *OUT/LOOK's* political and cultural agenda in a new format. We aim to revitalize a queer public sphere in which to explore questions that urgently concern all LGBTQ communities. The movement that started with Stonewall was built on the struggles for political and civil rights of people of color, women, labor unions, and the disabled. These struggles led, unwittingly, to a major reconfiguration of the sex/gender system. The world of Stonewall was fading, and the new queer world was being born.

Our first books in this series address themes of queering consent, queer archive interventions, and whether PrEP is a pill for promiscuity. Each book finds a way to dive into the deep nuances and discomforts of each topic. Other books on the struggle for an LGBTQ K-12 curriculum, the intersection of race and gender, transgenerational performance, and the incarceration of people with AIDS are in preparation.

We anticipate future volumes on shifting lesbian, queer, and trans identities; immigration, race, and homophobia; queer aging and the future of queer communities; new forms of community-based queer history; and LGBTQ politics after marriage, to name a few. Each book features multiple points of view, strong art, and a strong editorial concept.

In this era of new political dangers, Q+ Public takes on the challenges we face and offers a forum for public dialogue. AIDS changed the social context of sex for gay men, and many of us clearly felt that sex in general, after the advent of AIDS, offered potentially less pleasure and more danger than before. The epidemic instilled a profound sense of paranoia about homosexual desire. *A Pill for Promiscuity* tackles the historical weight of HIV/AIDS and recent pharmaceutical promises of freedom embedded into contemporary gay men's sexual cultures. The chapters in this collection feature a variety of genres, including memoir, ethnography and theory, manifesto, dialogue, and graphic comics. We hope you find them moving, exciting, and provocative.

E. G. Crichton
Jeffrey Escoffier

A Pill for Promiscuity

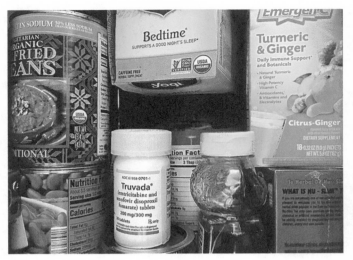

Ted Kerr, *Still-Life with Truvada*, 2021. Inspired by artist Joey Terill's painting series *Still-Life*, which began in 1997, soon after life-saving medication became available, and continued to 2012, with the FDA's approval of Truvada as PrEP.

I see Truvada on bedside tables, in kitchen cupboards, and on shelves near the front door. I smile at these placements. It is intimate and illuminates the everydayness of HIV in many of our lives. I also find it frustrating. I think about my friends who hide their Biktarvy, Atripla, and Genvoya in sock drawers, in purposefully mislabeled pill bottles, and at the bottom of backpacks to keep their positive status from family, roommates, border agents, classmates, lovers, employers, cops, and friends. It's not that I want people to hide their PrEP. I just don't want anyone to have to hide their medication out of fear.

Introduction

Why Promiscuity Matters

ANDREW SPIELDENNER AND JEFFREY ESCOFFIER

Slut. Whore. Trash. Skank. All words to describe people presumed to be promiscuous. Not *loving, free-spirited,* or *connected with the community.* The words we have about sexual freedom are value-laden and often negative. Notions of morality undergird this choice of words, as if the pursuit of sex or being sexually open somehow marks a body as amoral, our character somehow "less than." Why can't we just enjoy sex?

Sex is important. At different parts of our lives—for some of us—sex is one way to organize our time. Some of us discovered places where we could get off—certain bars, clubs, streets, parks, bathrooms, and truck stops. We created online spaces and apps for the same purpose. Sex provides for physical, psychic, and spiritual needs. It can be a bridge to connect to another or to ourselves. It can also be the door that closes off other kinds of communication or relationship possibilities. Sex has been central to the gay community across the world as we have fought to decriminalize and depathologize gay sex.

As gay, bi, queer, and trans people, we have been shamed for our desire. As children, we are not encouraged to discuss these longings, much less pursue them. We do anyway, leading to awkward encounters and searches for knowledge: How do I do this? What feels good? What am I supposed to do? We develop routines, scripts about the roles we want to play, schemes to get what we want. And as we gain experience, these interests can change. Yet, still there is so little space to talk with others about the things that feel good, the things that don't, the many ways that we can measure satisfaction in our intimate connections—at least not in any meaningful or nuanced way.

Still, gay men have been synonymous in social discourse with promiscuity; we are associated with group sex, anonymous sex partners, bathhouses, fetish and kink, sex toys, and recreational party drugs. We are watched by police when we enter parks at night or go in certain parts of the city. In the media, we are often depicted as pedophiles or corrupters of youth. Porn industries recognize us as consumers: we have an entire market aimed at us. We have online sex sites available that make encounters quicker and more efficient than those aimed at our straight counterparts.

We have invented new sexual acts and publicly celebrate our current ones. We built our communities through our promiscuity; we made connections with people from different social classes, races, and ethnicities. We learned our history from different generations through our sexual connections. And, yes, we've even achieved intimacy through our promiscuous connections.[1] We use a dynamic language about our sex, with multiple acronyms and abbreviations that differ slightly on each website or app or in each neighborhood. Samuel Delany, in his remarkable memoir of promiscuous sex in the porn theaters of Times Square, even argues that the kinds of social spaces and forms of sociality pioneered by gay men should be considered as useful models for sexual interaction between men and women as well—and as he emphasized, for "all women, single, married, straight, gay, prostitute, or society matron."[2]

The sexual pride of gay men has been accompanied by (or resulted from) a historical community and institutional discrimination based on our sex lives and the perception of our "sluttiness." This discrimination has taken many forms, including blaming someone for their HIV or sexually transmitted infection (STI) diagnosis as if they deserved it. It has also meant an ongoing criminalization of gay men in the areas of public sex and HIV.

For us, HIV changed the social context of sex: many of us strongly felt that sex in general, after the advent of HIV, offered potentially less pleasure and more danger than before. The epidemic instilled a profound sense of paranoia about homosexual desire. Was the sex that we engaged in—particularly, anal intercourse and the possibility of multiple orgasms with many partners—"inherently" dangerous or bad? Could gay men continue to engage in sex at all if it meant risking death from HIV? How could gay men have sex in the midst of an epidemic of a deadly sexually transmitted disease?[3] Many observers attributed the outbreak to sexual promiscuity and the frequent patronage of bathhouses and other public sex venues. Many physicians, epidemiologists, and social critics (both inside and outside the gay male community) urged gay men to stop having sex.[4] But abstaining from sex completely was obviously not a long-term option. After a period of uncertainty and confusion—about the cause of the immunodeficiency, what could prevent its spread, and how it could be treated—the knowledge that it was blood-borne and could be spread through sexual intercourse (anal and vaginal) suggested a partial solution: use of a condom.[5]

Gay, bisexual, queer, and trans people had to learn to engage in safer sex to prevent the acquisition or transmission of the disease. It was gay men, facing the demand to stop having sex, who went on to develop safer sex guidelines. These guidelines allowed gay men to engage in a wide variety of sex acts and remain fairly confident that they would neither transmit the disease nor acquire it. At some point a community consensus formed around condom use. The specter of the disease, with its massive death toll and impact in the LGBTQ community, haunts many of us, whether we contracted it or not, whether we knew someone who had died from it or not.[6] Two decades of prevention messages made "use a condom" a mantra in the gay community. Every gay sex act was enacted under the rule of the condom—its use or non-use labeling it "safe" or "risky." There are generations of gay men who used a condom for oral sex and anal sex and others who chose other ways to manage risk.

Often this "safer sex" meant to use a condom for every sex act with a man; sometimes it meant to reduce the number of sexual partners or the kinds of substances one used when sexing. The "safer sex" discourse often overproscribed anal sex. The focus on condom use, and its usage in anal penetration, closed off discussions of oral sex, frottage, bondage, fisting, or other activities that did not require a condom to prevent the transmission or acquisition of HIV.

Several scientific breakthroughs converged in the gay community to change this discourse. One was the discovery that a person living with HIV who is virologically suppressed cannot pass the disease to anyone else. Another, more commercialized breakthrough was the emergence of HIV *Pre-Exposure Prophylaxis* (PrEP), a once-daily medication that prevents disease acquisition. If you are HIV-negative and you take PrEP, you will likely remain that way regardless of condom use. In different parts of the world, PrEP is also available as an episodic intervention (rather than daily) and as a long-term injectable. In the United States, PrEP use has been pushed to the gay community through commercials, doctors' advice, community health initiatives, public health campaigns, and social media and influencers. PrEP and viral suppression even moved barebacking or raw sex from the fringe of gay pornography to the norm.

Silencing Sex

Within the gay community, respectability politics tends toward anti-sex, demanding a heteronormative appearance that includes monogamy and the possibility of marriage while excluding everything else. Within this frame, individuals should not engage in varieties of sex, much less talk about it. The cheerfulness of respectability politics belies its shame about both sex and the uncomfortable truths found in physical intimacy.

Our sex lives have loomed large in public health and clinical medicine. For four decades, gay sex has been intimately involved in one of the most devastating global epidemics of the twentieth century. There are extensive studies in HIV epidemiology in the rates of STIs and HIV across race and age. Public health researchers have examined the number of partners we have, the reasons we have for using a condom, the kinds of substances we imbibe, and the places we have had sex. Clinicians are concerned about the number of STIs or the presence of HIV or our use of prescriptions for erectile enhancers. Researchers have been less concerned with pleasure, desire, or context in the course of gay sex.

For four decades, the gay community has promoted "safer sex" to prevent the transmission or acquisition of HIV.[7] The effect of the trauma of HIV has been double-edged. On the one hand, HIV and the problematics of transmission and prevention have educated the public and even gay men about gay sexuality, especially anal intercourse (at a level, completely unimaginable before HIV). Yet, on the other hand, the preeminence of the political battles over gay marriage has obscured why promiscuity matters. It has encouraged a kind of domestication of homosexual eroticism and its incorporation into marital scripts.

Barebacking became a social concern in the 1990s and 2000s. Gay men who barebacked used multiple codes in online screen names to facilitate this interaction, such as "BB" or "raw." Websites specific to this sexual act emerged. In some circles, barebacking signified the presence of HIV, and people who engaged in barebacking were considered "sluts" and uncaring in their relationship to the gay community.

Unmasking the Sex

After we started editing this book, the COVID-19 pandemic hit, and most of us spent more than a year in some kind of social isolation, wearing a mask and reducing travel. COVID-19 again showed how ill prepared the government is to manage pandemics. Yet gay, bisexual, and other queer men were already accustomed to living in a pandemic, negotiating health risks, and understanding the importance of data protection and the harms of criminalization. The COVID-19 pandemic reminded us of the importance of unmediated interaction. We are wary again of strangers; we are trying to find new ways to have sex under new rules that frown on random, multiple partners. If we break those rules—whether by traveling or having sex—we cannot tell most of our friends, family, or even social media for fear of shaming, both privately and publicly. How do we manage the need for touch? We still have to imagine promiscuity.

Monkey Pox brings us another moment where public health is unsure of how to approach gay sex. The disease began to appear unexpectedly mostly amongst gay men, at first in Europe and Canada, then in other countries. Public health is struggling to come out with messaging and interventions that are useful, effective, and not homophobic. Questions around promiscuity again abound—with different countries and regions having varying approaches. Canada has supplied a vaccine to gay, bi, queer, and trans people for free, primarily working with sexual health centers and bathhouses. As of 2022, other countries are short on vaccine, and have not started working with community centers in the same way. Some have even taken the opportunity to further marginalize gay, bi, trans, and queer people.

PrEP and viral suppression have given gay, bisexual, and other queer folks the possibility to engage in sex without a condom without the fear of HIV. For the first time in decades, our community is not shaming people for not using condoms. *BB*, *raw*, *cum guzzler*, *cum dump*—these do not seem to carry the same moral judgment as other terms about promiscuity, at least not now. PrEP and its promise of viral suppression have presented pharmaceutical solutions to unmediated physical connections.

With this tool, most public health agencies have been talking about the "end of HIV" and have put forward plans to achieve that goal. The concept of ending the HIV epidemic, while laudable and a welcome respite from decades of crisis, does not seem possible, at least in the current political and economic moment—when gay and bisexual men, transgender people, people who use drugs, and sex workers are the majority of new HIV diagnoses globally and remain criminalized, stigmatized, and discriminated against in most of the world.

These prevention pills are not an easy solution. They require access and affordability: people not only have to want to use them but also be able to use them. Although taking a pill once a day does not seem burdensome, both of us can tell you that taking daily medications is demanding. It reminds one of ill health, it can interrupt the flow of the day, and there are days where other things are going on and the pill box goes untouched. Both of us manage daily med regimes for a range of conditions brought on by aging and other health conditions.

Neither of us has used a condom since the late 1990s and early 2000s, respectively. We did this for different reasons. Our sexual lives changed as we got older and became less concerned with anal sex. Andrew seroconverted and chose to pursue partners mostly living with HIV. Jeffrey entered his sixties and seventies and, in general, had less sex. Our practices had little to do with PrEP or viral suppression: rather we had individual journeys that did not necessitate condoms.

There are other pills for promiscuity such as those for erectile dysfunction, hormone treatments, and substances like Molly or Ecstasy that alter moods and sensations. Even birth control pills have been painted with the promiscuity brush. This book comes out of a recognition that gay, bisexual, queer, and trans men are encountering the discourse of promiscuity within the context of pharma. We were curious how these pharmaceutical interventions are understood and practiced.

The collection of voices here reminds us a little of a conversation we might have had on the outside patio of the Metropolitan, one of Brooklyn's oldest bars. It would have been a mixed crowd. Some older guys. A bunch of younger guys too. Academics, activists, writers, and artists, but regular folks as well. As the conversation turned to the impact of PrEP on our sex lives and how it seemed to encourage an increase in casual sex, the talk would become more raucous. One of the older men at the gathering would be author Andrew Holleran, back in the city for a short visit. His book, *Dancer from the Dance*, published in 1978, is a bestselling novel set on Fire Island and among the circuit parties and discotheques of New York: it captured the frenetic gay world of sex, romance, and dancing during the 1970s. In 1988, he published *Ground Zero*, a collection of essays, originally appearing in *Christopher Street* magazine, that offered a broad assessment of gay life before and during the early years of the AIDS epidemic. His "Notes on Promiscuity" (reprinted here as chapter 1) was one of those essays. He starts off this book by reminding us of all the different ways to understand promiscuity.

Cartoonist Steve MacIsaac speaks for all the young men who came out during the early and most devastating years of the epidemic. To become a sexually active gay man during the 1980s and 1990s, it was necessary to confront the fear of HIV and discover the pleasures and excitement of sex. MacIsaac is an award-winning comics artist, known for his *Shirtlifter* series (vols. 1–6, 2006–2019), which explores gay men's relationships and lives, especially their sex and sexuality. He is "interested in how sex defines people and how it can be a sublime way of revealing character and motivation. People let their guard down when you sleep with them; you often get to know them in a way that doesn't happen when you're simply friends. I think that's one reason why, for gay men, sex is so often a path to or conduit for building friendships."[8] He is joined in the book by Daniel Felsenthal, a music writer for *Pitchfork* and an art critic for the *Village Voice*, who writes about books, movies, LGBT life and history, and all sorts of personal stuff, as well as fiction. Gay activist and writer, Alex Garner, might be holding court nearby, proudly explaining the multiple possibilities of gay and poz life in his second home in Mexico City.

But what about PrEP and sex? Kane Race, from Australia, discusses what puzzles him about the initial reluctance of many gay men to use PrEP. Nic Flores and Deion Hawkins join the conversation with their perspectives of their personal lives and the challenges faced by their respective communities of color to gain access to and use PrEP; they also address how sex has to be relearned. All three are university-based academics, tightly connected to the people and places that comprise their communities—and as likely to be found in a gay bar as a classroom. Pornographic film director Mister Pam extends the discussion to how people in gay sex-work industries have experienced PrEP and the many tests and conversations that become unnecessary.

Addison Vawters critiques the ways that pharmaceutical industries have become ubiquitous in our lives, claiming to extend or improve any and all potential conditions related to the body and mind. A community-based scholar, Addison questions the costs and identities that these pharmacological interventions incur, encourage, and require. Lore/tta LeMaster discusses sex and pleasure at the intersections of gender, furthering the potentiality of erotics. How can one feel good in a body when our physique is constantly pushed into normative shapes? What are ways that we can free ourselves? Two more pieces explore notions of liberation: Ariel Sabillon looks at healing and trauma, as well as the role of sex in moving forward, and Justice Jamal Jones and coeditor Andrew Spieldenner engage in a dialogue about summoning each other and growth in a pandemic.

A Pill for Promiscuity is a collection of gay and queer folks imagining sex, and the many interactions leading up to it, in this moment. We writers and artists do not have a shared agreement about the value of promiscuity or pharmaceuticals. We do not have common gender or sexual identities. Some are gay, others bi, and still others are queer: some identify with being a man, and others are transitioning or are somewhere else on the gender spectrum. Our reference to "gay" in this book is similar to the best kind of gay bars—like 1990s El Rio on a Sunday afternoon deep in San Francisco's Mission—where a hodgepodge of people could and would show up, regardless of sexuality, sex, race, age, and socioeconomic status. Some were high, others sober; some were just starting their days, and others were getting there from last night. The culture was about community; the music was global. It was a kind of utopia: perfect moments before grinding back to work, rent, bills, family, partners, any number of obligations that constitute life in capitalism.

Notes

1. Etienne Meunier and Jeffrey Escoffier, "The Triumph of Collective Intimacy: Gay Collective Sex in New York City from the Late 1800s to Today," in *The Gayborhood Studies Reader: From Sexual Liberation to Cosmopolitan Spectacle*, ed. Christopher Conner and Daniel Okamura (Lanham, MD: Lexington Books, 2021), 85–105; Etienne Meunier, "Organizing Collective Intimacy: An Ethnography of New York's Clandestine Sex Clubs" (PhD diss., Rutgers University, 2016).

2. Samuel Delany, *Times Square Red, Times Square Blue*, 20th anniversary edition with a new foreword by Robert Reid-Pharr (New York: New York University Press, 2019), xvii, 197.

3. Douglas Crimp, "How to Have Promiscuity in an Epidemic?" in *AIDS: Cultural Analysis, Cultural Activism* (Cambridge, MA: MIT Press, 1987), 237–271; William G. Hawkeswood, *One of the Children: Gay Black Men in Harlem* (Berkeley: University of California, 1996), 169–184; Sonja Mackenzie, *Structural Intimacies:*

Sexual Stories in the Black AIDS Epidemic (New Brunswick, NJ: Rutgers University Press, 2013); Rafael M. Diaz, *Latino Gay Men and HIV: Culture, Sexuality and Risk Behavior* (New York: Routledge, 1998), 137–150.

4. The most prominent of these critics inside the gay male community was Larry Kramer, "1,112 and Counting," *New York Native*, March 14–27, 1983. See also his *Reports from the Holocaust: The Making of An AIDS Activist* (New York: St. Martin's Press, 1989).

5. Jeffrey Escoffier, "The Invention of Safer Sex: Vernacular Knowledge, Gay Politics, and HIV Prevention," *Berkeley Journal of Sociology* 43 (Spring 1999): 1–30.

6. World Health Organization, Global Health Observatory, https://www.who.int/data/gho/data/themes/hiv-aids#:~:text =Global%20situation%20and%20trends%3A,at%20othe%20 end%20of%202020.

7. Jeffrey Escoffier, "Sex, Safety and the Trauma of AIDS," *Women's Studies Quarterly* 39, nos. 1/2 (Spring/Summer 2011): 129–138.

8. Steven Surman, Steve MacIsaac/Comic Book Creator Interview, https://www.stevensurman.com/steve-macisaac-comic-book -creator-interview/.

1

Notes on Promiscuity, 1988

ANDREW HOLLERAN

Andrew Holleran, author of "Notes on Promiscuity," also wrote *Dancer from the Dance*, a best-selling novel set on Fire Island and among the circuit parties and discotheques of New York City that captured the frenetic gay world of sex, romance, and dancing. In 1988, he published *Ground Zero*, a collection of essays that originally appeared in *Christopher Street* magazine. "Notes on Promiscuity" was one of those essays that offered a broad assessment of gay life before and during the early years of the AIDS epidemic. It is reprinted here from *Ground Zero* with permission (New York: New American Library, 1988).

1. If a young man is promiscuous, we say he is *sowing his oats*; if a young woman is promiscuous, we say she is a *slut*; if a homosexual of any age is promiscuous, we say he is a *neurotic example of low self-esteem*.
2. Everyone has his/her own definition of promiscuity.
3. A person who is promiscuous professionally is a prostitute. Most people who are promiscuous would be shocked if

you called them a prostitute, however, because they do not think of themselves that way, simply because they do not charge money.

4. There is a tribe of people in Uganda so promiscuous that the name of the tribe is also the word for prostitute.

5. Promiscuity is thought of in two ways: as having many, many different partners and as having no standards for the people with whom one sleeps. The second type is comparatively rare, however, and is held in contempt by the first. The worst thing we can say about someone is that he/she will sleep with *anybody*.

6. But the truth is that many of us will sleep with *almost* anybody.

7. In ancient Rome, a certain empress would slip out of the palace at night, Juvenal tells us, to take a room in a local brothel and entertain customers until dawn. This was being both promiscuous *and* a prostitute. (*And* bored.) (*And* an empress.)

8. Sex is a pleasurable experience repeated many, many times during our lives that, if experienced with the same person each time, is considered responsible, adult, mature; if experienced with a different person each time, it is considered promiscuous.

9. Americans, products of a consumer society, with a short attention span, a bent for instant gratification inculcated by advertising, and a fairly lonesome society, are made for promiscuity. Some gay men think promiscuity is a revolutionary ideal that can transform the world, release human energy, and make the planet a better place to live.

10. Others think promiscuity is the freeway to hell.

11. It takes time to become promiscuous. Married couples reading stories about AIDS are astounded to learn that a homosexual man has slept with eight hundred men; to the homosexual reader, this does not seem that bizarre.

12. The word for promiscuity in gay life is "tricking."

13. Tricking depends on motive—one may not consider oneself promiscuous at all, for instance, though at the end of ten years of tricking you've slept with many people.

14. (Once, when someone asked me, "Do you consider yourself promiscuous?" I realized that though I'd slept with a number of different people, I had never considered myself promiscuous.)

15. Before the plague, promiscuity was a growth industry.

16. Before the plague, promiscuity was the sore point of homosexual life. Why—even gay men wish to know—did homosexuals convert liberation into promiscuity?

17. No one knows.

18. When a friend asked me, "Why are gay men promiscuous?" I started to reply, "Because they don't marry and have children, because they feel guilty about being gay, because they're men, because men are like dogs, because they're lonely, because everyone would have as much sex as he could if he could, because sex is the most transcendent experience"—then I saw my friend lighting another cigarette, and I said, "Why do you smoke?"

19. Promiscuity was the lingua franca, the Esperanto, of the male homosexual community.

20. Men are now weeping in doctors' offices over the fact that they were once promiscuous.

21. Men are now telling other men in the new cities they've moved to that they never were promiscuous.

22. (Gay men now suspect each other of promiscuity.)

23. Gay men have been blamed for the plague by people who say promiscuity caused AIDS.

24. But promiscuity flourished in the seventies precisely because it *was* disease-free (or so everyone thought). That is, every disease acquired via promiscuous sex was curable with some form of penicillin.

25. In fact, promiscuity's considerable charm may be measured by the number of afflictions people were willing to put up with as the *occupational hazards* of promiscuity. Until AIDS, these were crabs, scabies, venereal warts, syphilis, gonorrhea, anal fissures, amoebiasis, hepatitis, and (the first one to give promiscuous heterosexuals pause) herpes.

26. Once, while leaving the public health clinic on Ninth Avenue, I asked a friend how he was going to celebrate the test results that showed he had finally rid himself of intestinal parasites, and he replied, "By going to the Mineshaft tonight." Such was the allure of promiscuity.

27. Promiscuity is now inseparable from the dread of AIDS.

28. Yet promiscuity must be separated from the issue of AIDS if one wants to evaluate it, because no one in the past was promiscuous knowing it would lead to what it led to.

29. People were promiscuous in the past for a simple reason: "Sexual practices are banal, impoverished, doomed to repetition," Roland Barthes said, "and this impoverishment is disproportionate to the wonder of the pleasure they afford."

30. And: "I have spoken of pleasure," wrote Renaud Camus in his introduction to *Tricks*, "but I don't see what . . . would keep me from calling such moments happiness."

31. And: "How can we not desire, afterward, to encounter similar moments once again, even if only once more?"

32. *Once more* (or *Once Is Not Enough*) is the *mantra* of promiscuity.

33. The motto of promiscuity is *So Many Men, So Little Time.*

34. The slogan of promiscuity is *Show us your meat.*

35. Many celebrated people, including presidents, have been promiscuous—John F. Kennedy, for example.

36. Very few homosexual men are not or have never been promiscuous.

37. The nature of promiscuity came clear to me the night at the baths when I looked back at the doorway of the room whose occupant I had just fallen deeply in love with after the most wonderful, intense, earth-shattering, intimate, and ecstatic sex and watched another man walk into his room and close the door behind him with a little click.

38. Promiscuity offends that deep desire W. H. Auden said was not merely to be loved, but "to be loved alone."

39. Promiscuity entails a double standard: we want to be promiscuous ourselves, but we want the people we sleep with to want only us.

40. The average person thinks other people have sex with him because he is good-looking, sexy, special, attractive. In a promiscuous world, however, we are picked up mostly because we are *breathing* . . .

41. The first law of promiscuous physics is: Over a long enough period of time, everyone sleeps with everyone else.

42. The second law of promiscuous physics is: Every face is new to someone.

43. The third law of promiscuous physics is: The thousandth trick is not what the first one was.

44. There is no telling where promiscuity would have led homosexual men had the plague not occurred; it is possible it might have faded away, as people grew tired or disillusioned with it; or it is possible people would have started coming to work—as a friend predicted—"with broken arms."

45. When asked why he was moving from New York City to San Francisco in 1978, a friend of mine said with an ironic smile, "To improve the quality of my promiscuity."

46. He is now dead.

47. Tennessee Williams said, "Each time I pick someone up on the street, I leave a piece of my heart in the gutter."

48. Oscar Wilde said, "I lie in the gutter, but look up at the stars."

49. (Now that it is denied them, people realize how romantic promiscuity was.)

50. Promiscuity gave rise to two terms of gay slang: *fast food sex* and the *sex junky*.

51. No one can ever be sure why people are promiscuous.

52. One friend of mine said, "I had no choice but to be promiscuous—no one ever wanted to see me a second time."

53. Some people are promiscuous because they are looking for a lover.

54. Others are promiscuous because they have already found one.

55. Promiscuity anesthetizes many aches.

56. Promiscuity ups the ante with each sexual encounter.

57. Promiscuity is the nightmare of Don Juan.

58. Promiscuity is the quest for what can never be attained.

59. Promiscuity is hope.

60. Promiscuity is a sadness, a rut, a daily self-degradation.

61. Promiscuity is the last true adventure, the last ecstasy, the last *rainforest* of industrial-consumer man.

62. Promiscuity is a means of remaining a perpetual adolescent.

63. Promiscuity is a means of growing up.

64. Promiscuity fails to satisfy that most important need—for intimacy, rootedness, shelter.

65. Promiscuity supplies these in small, ecstatic doses.

66. Promiscuity is a sexual version of chain smoking.

67. Promiscuity is a sexual version of kneeling in church.

68. Promiscuity is a school of hard knocks, the parent that abuses all its children.

69. Promiscuity gives us something we can acquire no other way: the wisdom of prostitutes.

70. One effect of hiring a hustler, or paying for sex, is the realization afterward that sex is something most people will do with you for *nothing*! One night, after leaving a hustler's apartment in New York, on my way home, I walked through a park filled with men cruising and was startled to realize that all of them would do for free exactly what had just cost me thirty-five dollars.

71. Promiscuity squanders—one has nothing to show for years and years of spent sperm.

72. Promiscuity forms character, builds men.

73. Promiscuity is always planning its next expedition.

74. Promiscuity eventually degenerates into mere habit and, like any habit, is very hard to break.

75. Harder to break than, say, cigarette smoking, because promiscuity is an attempt to escape from loneliness.

76. Promiscuity guarantees loneliness.

77. Many people enjoy promiscuity in their prime and then denounce it in middle age. (Saint Augustine is the most famous of these.)

78. In youth, promiscuity bestows the rapture of poets and saints.

79. In old age, it means haunting the truck stops on I-75.

80. When the author of *Tricks* jokingly told one of his partners, "You know I only like you for your ass," the man replied, in total seriousness, "Yes, I know." (This funny, and sad, exchange sums up the nature of promiscuity.)

81. In a promiscuous world, people come to believe they are worth no more than their genitals.

82. In a promiscuous world, they're right.

83. When Henry James returned to visit America in 1910, he was struck by the great number of New Yorkers eating candy bars. Seventy years later, we were eating each other: the penis as lollipop.

84. It is pointless to feel guilty about promiscuity, so long as you enjoy(ed) it and harm(ed) no one. One may, after all, have brought joy into the lives of others, and it was, let's face it, a great adventure.

85. Almost everyone disdains promiscuity.

86. Yet all those who think abstinence will be practiced by the majority of people during the age of AIDS—all those who think promiscuity has ceased—are deluded.

87. As King Lear said, "Let copulation thrive; the gilded fly doth lecher in my sight."

88. (As Anthony said of Cleopatra, "She makes hungry where most she satisfies.")

89. It took three or four years for promiscuity to slow down to its present level, after the appearance of AIDS, for a simple reason: stopping promiscuity was like stopping Niagara Falls.

90. Promiscuity ceases the moment one falls in love.

91. It resumes when that condition fades.

92. Promiscuity was once associated with joy, travel, toothpaste, Brazil, San Juan, Paris, Berlin, hamburgers, automobiles, insurance, poppers, gymnasiums, designer jeans, designer drugs, Calvin Klein underwear, discotheques, cosmetics, vitamins. Clothes, movies, airplanes, subways, men's rooms, piers, Central Park, Land's End, Buena Vista Park, Folsom Street, the West Side Highway, marijuana, cocaine, ethyl chloride, Mexico, the Philippines, Miami, Provincetown, Fire Island, Canal Jeans, Bloomingdale's, the balcony of the Saint, bars, baths, sidewalks, Lisbon, Madrid, Mykonos, certain magazines, four A.M., Stuyvesant Park, the grocery store, the laundromat, autumn, summer, winter, spring, bicycles, T-shirts, and Rice-A-Roni.

93. Not anymore.

Perspective

Fear

The AIDS epidemic instilled a profound sense of paranoia about homosexual desire. "Sex is just a completely different thing now," porn star/director Al Parker exclaimed, "The entire time you're having sex you're thinking, 'I'm having sex with everybody this person ever had sex with. I wonder what he's done and where he's been and if he's positive or negative. I wonder if I'm giving him anything.' If you can keep a hard-on while all this is going on in your head, you're better than I am." Could gay men continue to engage in sex at all if it meant risking death? Before the development of effective HIV antiretroviral (ARV) therapies, HIV was considered a death sentence. The fear was so thick that governments created laws to criminalize sex and drug use for people living with HIV (so-called HIV criminalization laws), which remain on the books in many states and countries today. Celebrities openly expressed fear and disgust with people living with HIV.

Health departments, physicians, and even some leaders in the LGBTQ community encouraged gay men to stop having sex. Of course, most gay men thought that it would be difficult to stop, but many others, traumatized by the plague that had wiped out dozens of their friends, did stop having anal sex. They turned to porn or fantasy or tried to imagine a sex life consisting solely of kissing, embracing, and masturbation. After a period of uncertainty and confusion—about what caused the immunodeficiency, what could prevent its spread, and how it could be treated—the knowledge that it was blood-borne and could be spread through sexual intercourse (anal and vaginal) suggested a partial solution: use of a condom.

As condom use became the normative sexual practice in the late 1980s, the rates of HIV transmission in the United States dropped dramatically. However, by the mid-1990s they had plateaued. Initially the presumption was that unless you knew the other person's serostatus (once an HIV test became available), everyone else was HIV-positive. Yet, no norm, however well established, is followed 100 percent of the time. During the early nineties, there was a slow resurgence of sexual activity. Parallel to this resurgence was the development of new combination ARV therapies that contributed to the impression that HIV could be a manageable chronic condition, much like diabetes. Pharmaceutical firms reinforced that impression by running ads for these new drugs featuring healthy-looking, physically fit men climbing mountains. Rates for syphilis, which had fallen along with rates of HIV infection in the previous decade when the condom code prevailed, began to rise, provoking debate about "condom fatigue" and the impact on gay men's sexual health of new medications for HIV such as protease inhibitors, which were more effective than earlier treatments.

Public recognition of the impending crisis around safer sex surfaced in 1994. By the end of the nineties, the number of gay men who reported not using a condom (as well as those having sex with multiple partners) rose from 25 to 45 percent according to a 1999 study by the Centers for Disease Control and Prevention (CDC). In a 2003 CDC study in New York City, 55 percent of men reporting anal sex with another man had not used a condom. Porn star/writer Scott O'Hara announced that he was "tired of using condoms." HIV activist Stephen Gendin wrote of the thrill of not using condoms to have sex with other HIV-positive men. He explained that the term "barebacking" was derived from riding horseback without a saddle. Porn star Tony Valenzuela, in impromptu remarks made at a conference on gay community organizing, shared that the "erotic charge and intimacy I feel when a man comes inside me is transformational, especially in a climate which so completely disregards its importance." These comments were followed by similar admissions from gay journalist Michelangelo Signorile and queer theorist Michael Warner, signaling a crisis of what Gabriel Rotello called the "condom code." It was also in the early nineties that a "second wave" of HIV was observed.

For those gay, bisexual, and queer men who never knew a world without HIV, barebacking presented the opportunity to explore sexuality without layers between bodies. By the mid-1990s, there was some acceptance of HIV within the gay community: many were part of social support networks in which someone had seroconverted or worked for HIV organizations. Was the fear of HIV enough to keep another generation from getting HIV?

In 2012 a "pre-exposure prophylaxis" (abbreviated as PrEP) was developed by Gilead Sciences to prevent transmission of HIV to individuals who are HIV- negative. PrEP was an offshoot of research by pharmaceutical companies that produced treatments for those who were HIV-positive.

It currently requires taking a daily pill, although other forms of PrEP (i.e., long-acting injections) are being developed. Although many governments and health organizations have promoted the adoption of PrEP to help reduce rates of HIV, it is opposed by critics who believe it encourages risky or promiscuous sexual behavior.

2
Safe

STEVE MACISAAC

SAFE - an introduction

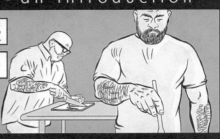

THE WEIRDEST THING ABOUT BEING AN AUTOBIOGRAPHICAL CARTOONIST IS SEEING YOUR LIFE BECOME A HISTORICAL ARTIFACT.

I STARTED MAKING COMICS TO FIGURE OUT THE GAY COMMUNITY. I WAS HAVING A HARD TIME FINDING MY PLACE WITHIN IT.

I CAME OUT PRETTY LATE: TWENTY-SIX.

FEAR OF INFECTION PLAYED NO SMALL PART IN THE DELAY.

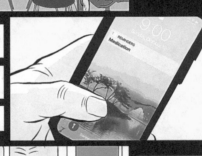

I BOUGHT MY FIRST BODYBUILDING MAGAZINE IN 1984. MY FIRST TIME MASTURBATING TO A PICTURE OF AN ALMOST NAKED MAN.

I LEARNED ABOUT AIDS THE SAME YEAR. A DIFFERENT MAGAZINE. *ROLLING STONE.*

BY THE TIME I GOT A GIRLFRIEND AND BECAME SEXUALLY ACTIVE, AIDS WAS VERY WELL KNOWN, EVEN IN SMALL TOWN CANADA.

MY CATHOLIC UNIVERSITY EVEN BROUGHT IN YOUNG PEOPLE WHO HAD BECOME POSITIVE, ALL OF THEM HETEROSEXUAL.

IN MY HEAD, IF EVEN STRAIGHT PEOPLE COULD GET IT, THEN GAYS HAD ZERO CHANCE.

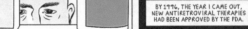

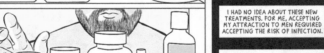

BY 1996, THE YEAR I CAME OUT, NEW ANTIRETROVIRAL THERAPIES HAD BEEN APPROVED BY THE FDA.

I HAD NO IDEA ABOUT THESE NEW TREATMENTS. FOR ME, ACCEPTING MY ATTRACTION TO MEN REQUIRED ACCEPTING THE RISK OF INFECTION.

CONTINUED DENIAL, THE CERTAINTY OF DEPRESSION AND ANHEDONIA.

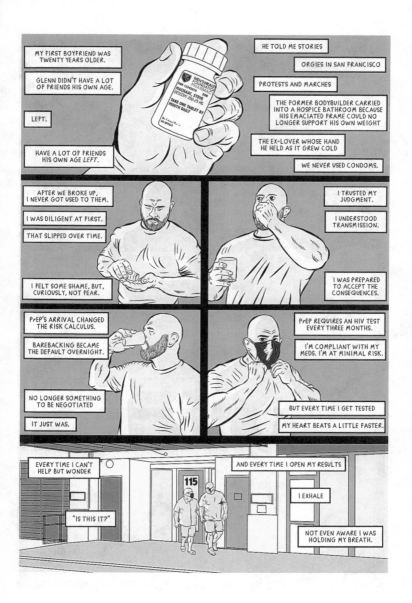

S A F E

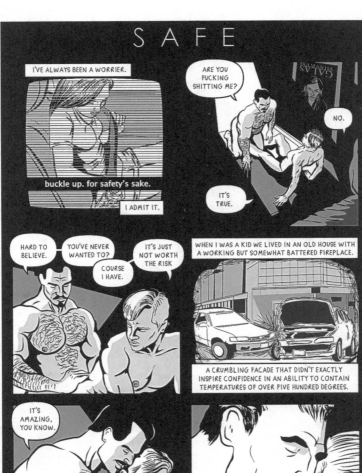

I'VE ALWAYS BEEN A WORRIER.

buckle up. for safety's sake.

I ADMIT IT.

ARE YOU FUCKING SHITTING ME?

NO.

IT'S TRUE.

HARD TO BELIEVE.

YOU'VE NEVER WANTED TO?

COURSE I HAVE.

IT'S JUST NOT WORTH THE RISK

WHEN I WAS A KID WE LIVED IN AN OLD HOUSE WITH A WORKING BUT SOMEWHAT BATTERED FIREPLACE.

A CRUMBLING FACADE THAT DIDN'T EXACTLY INSPIRE CONFIDENCE IN AN ABILITY TO CONTAIN TEMPERATURES OF OVER FIVE HUNDRED DEGREES.

IT'S AMAZING, YOU KNOW.

HMPH.

FOR YOU, MAYBE.

FOR YOU, TOO.

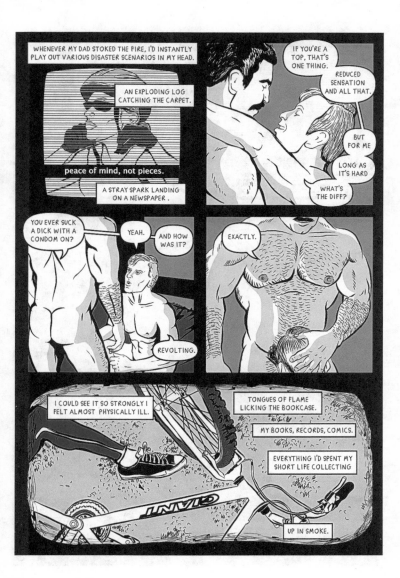

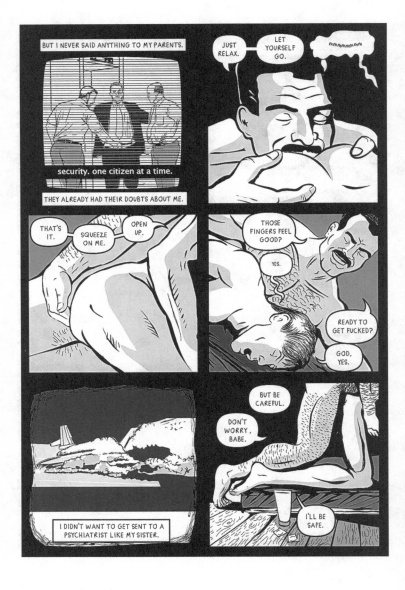

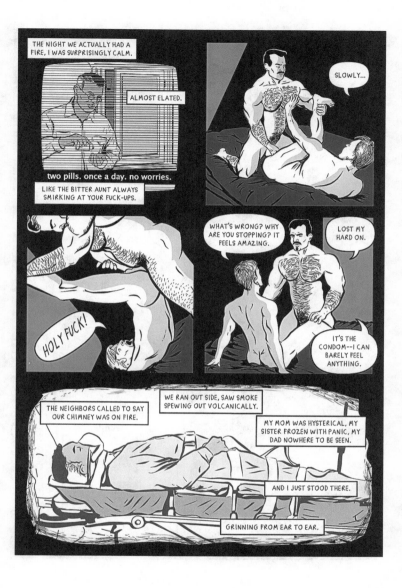

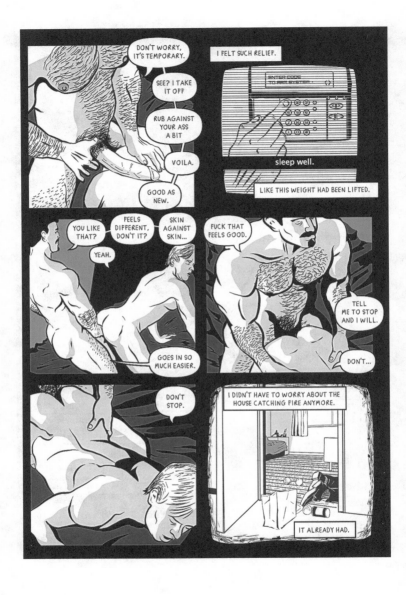

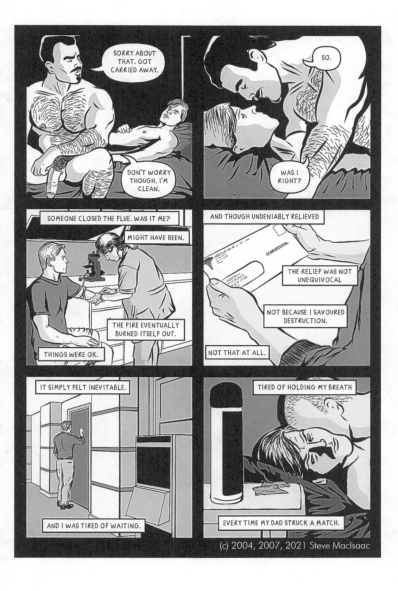

3

How I Learned to Stop Worrying, or the Straight Panic Defense

DANIEL FELSENTHAL

When it came to health, my first memories were of panic. I wiped my ass too hard, found blood on the tissue, and thought I had colon cancer. I touched a swollen lymph node—and my eight-year-old self was sure I was afflicted with the Black Death. In the context of my family, this frenzied behavior was ordinary: my mother, saddled with raising three children while also working, was an utter panic queen. One summer, my sister came back from sleepaway camp with head lice, and mom spearheaded preventive measures so relentless they make today's mask wearer look like a COVID denier. Never again could I borrow a coat, wear a pinny in gym class, or hang an article of clothing in a closet at a friend's place: any of these acts might bring dreaded pests into our household.

I tended to panic because I believed I was cause for panic. Quarrelsome and disobedient, I questioned everything my parents said until they became incensed. One day, I returned from school to find mom pale, looking grave. She'd been diagnosed with macular degeneration, a thinning in the retina that causes vision loss. The condition was stress-induced, and I was the most stressful person around. "You have to stop fighting with me because you're making me go blind." The doctor, we learned later, had misdiagnosed her; instead, she had a far less serious condition. But being blamed for someone else's illness stuck in my craw. Clearly, it's still there today.

When I grew up in the 1990s and 2000s, AIDS was just beginning to be something other than a death sentence—for those who were privileged enough to afford drugs. The only queer I knew during early childhood, my uncle, was also cause for panic. He had been outed (dramatically, of course!) when his wife walked in on him having sex with another man. He was an addict—of marijuana—he told my parents, who equated weed with heroin because they believed that he was telling the truth. One Thanksgiving, he and dad fought because my uncle used my father's razor blade to shave. Of course, dad could have washed the implement with soap and hot water, yet it was 1996, and gay blood provoked hysteria. We kids learned a clear lesson: anxiety should always crowd out reason, bullying it to the margins with self-righteous purpose.

My uncle's "risky" lifestyle often made him seem like my parents' polar opposite. In fact, he was also a sufferer of panic. Several years ago, he died after trying to ignore a stomachache by dosing himself with crystal meth and pills; he turned out to have a routine case of appendicitis. Panicking can lead to failing to take deliberate steps toward self-protection. It's an emotion, and you can tap into terror and be just as ineffectual as someone who is totally care-free—with preventable conditions to show for your pain.

On my twenty-first birthday, the Federal Drug Administration authorized Truvada as an HIV-preventive medication.

Though I was having sex with men at the time, largely in "risky" settings such as back rooms, I didn't take the drug for a number of years. My goal was not good health, but instead to avoid seeing doctors, who I believed were capable only of tripping the wires of my inherited hysteria. Once, when I was a college freshman, I jerked off and looked down at my cumshot to find flecks of red in my semen. *I shot blood out of my dick.* The dread was immediate, fatalistic, consuming. Of course, I couldn't tell anyone what happened, certainly not a medical professional. I spun in place for days, hardly able to do my homework. Every couple of hours, I masturbated joylessly onto a sheet of printer paper and searched my semen for color. It stayed off-white, and I eased back into being an undergraduate.

My parents were always characters in my head, saying, *I would never live the same way as you; it's unsafe.* I'm sure my uncle suffered from similarly disapproving voices, and neither of us took the measured, sensible steps that might have made our risk-taking something other than a nihilistic denial of danger. The first time I had sex with several people in one day, I went to a heterosexual friend's house and confessed in terror: I was sure that I had caught something terminal. "You won't get AIDS now, in 2013," he told me calmly. "But of course, it is possible to get HIV."

My means of remaining seronegative were based on intuition, judgment, and semi-ersatz notions of how the virus is spread. Bottoming, I almost always used protection; if I topped, I hardly ever put on a condom. The major tenet of my "sexual health plan" was shunning poz people as partners, a behavior that I now see as unenlightened and discriminatory, as though I were a straight man a generation earlier hugging a gay friend and noticing in horror a cut on the homo's cheek. I asked people to reveal their HIV statuses in a manner that must have been more officious than sensitive.

Thanks to Grindr and Scruff, I knew the meaning of "Unde-tectable," but my knee-jerk sense of caution prevented me from even considering sleeping with men whose low viral loads made them untransmittable. The consequences of my prohibitory lifestyle were not medical, but social and spiritual. For years, I blinkered myself to a huge swatch of the gay world. My loss.

By using the mores of earlier generations to determine whom I should sleep with, rather than the science available to me in the twenty-first century, I was contributing to a culture of ignorance surrounding HIV. My virus education had been cobbled together from advertisements featuring Magic Johnson, high school sex ed, and conversations with doctors when I got tested; it was based around preventing me from getting the disease by making me afraid of its consequences. I was never taught about life as a seroconverted person. Visits to the doctor's office were unconcerned with fostering empathy between neg patients and those who had a stigmatic virus—rather, these experiences were a crash course in fleeing pleasure. Physicians and social workers interrogated me about my sexual, drinking, and drug habits. Did I like to rim ass? Don't I know that hepatitis is often spread through mouth-to-anus contact? How about sucking dick? Do I use a condom when I give head? (Umm, def no.) What about drinking? How many a night? My lifestyle and culture were invisible to them, as was my emotional response to being quizzed. The focus was on making patients believe that penetration, intoxication, and sodomy formed an unholy trinity of evil. "Wear a condom," they said, but their tone told me, "Abstinence only."

During these appointments, I flirted with being the complete worrywart I was as a child. Some might think that all this agonizing would motivate me to take PReP. Yet again, what I feared was not disease but instead the fear that the medical establishment instilled in me. In my early and mid-twenties, to see a doctor every three months to keep my prescription filled was unimaginable. All the doctors had to give me was shame.

However damaging scare-tactic preventive medicine may have been to my psyche, it's worse for the poz community, as well as for people with other STIs, turning them into bogeymen who might as well already be dead. Look up "herpes simplex" on MayoClinic.com, and you'll learn that HSV-2 is not only incurable but that it also can be contagious when sores are not present. The Mayo Clinic proposes an unrealistic prevention strategy: "Abstain from sexual activity or limit sexual contact to only one person who is infection-free." No need to mention that the chance of transmitting herpes when you don't have an outbreak is infinitesimal and that the possibility of being infectious only decreases as time goes on. A couple of my regular sexual partners contracted the virus decades ago, haven't had symptoms in years, and never infected me. I've also had partners who live in abject terror of herpes, treating the word "incurable" like a bloody scab they can't stop scratching. Both are victims of a medical system that prizes instilling individual fear over fostering healthy communities, leading us to blame and hate the ill.

Our response, however, should never be to shun health care but rather to learn how to navigate it without resorting to hysteria. Ironically, a great benefit of PrEP is that it forces me to go to the doctor. Since I started on Truvada, I have had some guilt-inducing conversations with physicians. Scared-shitless prevention strategies still exist in the realm of sexual medicine; no system is without its pain-in-the-ass moralists. Yet STI testing has become a trimonthly habit, as well as an unexpected lesson in how to navigate health without indulging panic. The experience has drawn the onus of sexual health away from the ceaseless spiral of *me* and toward the world at large. I take PrEP for the same reason that I wear a mask or get a COVID-19 vaccine—to work toward the end of a lethal, destructive epidemic. At the clinic, I think, I'm not sick, I haven't missed any pills, and I don't need to be here today. I showed up because I want to fight AIDS.

COVID-19 has put public health initiatives in the spotlight and introduced to many the concept that epidemiology is often diametrically opposed to hypochondria: it doesn't encourage varied responses to extreme fear but rather standardized, evolving methods that involve entire populations. These initiatives focus on saving the most lives possible, which undermines so many of the grossest aspects of our for-profit health care system, revealing how a solipsistic approach to battling illness can only be catastrophic. To take a macro example, the United States is rich enough to buy vaccine doses ad infinitum. Still, Americans will be in danger until the whole world manages to inoculate itself. The only option is to coordinate across borders and cultures—of course, humanity will fail, but although a future global initiative may be a practical disaster, it will still be a beacon of hope for humanism. Now we know for sure that the self-centeredness of twentieth-century life will only doom us in the future.

In many western nations, the era between World War II and 2020 was an historical outlier, because people, at least heterosexuals, could live largely without making communal sacrifices, never considering the possibility that they might have to temper their personal ambitions for the benefit of society. We have all learned from this mentality—too much. But queers know what it means to change your lifestyle for a greater good. We can set examples, leading the wolves who used to hunt us as though they're docile sheep. Unlike most heterosexuals, we've spent adulthood learning how to manage risk without closing ourselves to life's pleasures. Instead of splitting us apart, our shared outrage about sickness solidified homosexuality into a stronger community. Virus is not only an enemy to fight, we discovered: it's also a reality to live with.

Here are some helpful pointers, which I've inherited through the bloodlines of my progenitors in barebacking faggotry: Panic doesn't help. You won't get anywhere acting like a crazy queen. As for isolation? It can work for a while, but we know from experience that sitting in a closet-sized room, sad and alone, makes a person desperate. Life is still out there for us to enjoy, even improve. Just remember: everyone is dangerous, so no one is *dangerous*.

Perspective

Sex

It is now more than forty years since the discovery of HIV/AIDS. Since then, the ravages of the epidemic have swept the world—with an estimated 37.7 million people infected and currently living with HIV in 2020. Initially discovered among gay men in North America, the disease continues to have a huge impact throughout the world.

The epidemic provoked a devastating crisis—one that was political, cultural, and sexual. For homosexual men, AIDS was a historical trauma that shattered the experience of sexual freedom and disrupted new patterns of identity and community. In addition to the individual devastation caused by a mysterious and novel disease striking down hundreds of one's friends and fellow community members, critical personal, social, and clinical issues soon emerged: diminished erotic desire, increased sexual dysfunctions, sexual addiction, and declining participation in community institutions.

The impending epidemic provoked debate and conflict over what aspects of the "gay lifestyle"—relating either to sexual practices or recreational drug use—might have contributed to the pattern of immune deficiency among gay men. Many observers attributed the outbreak to sexual promiscuity, the frequent patronage of bathhouses and other public sex venues, and the general availability of sexual activity in the urban centers of San Francisco and New York. The "lifestyle" argument had dramatic public health implications. It suggested that prevention could only be achieved by modifying the whole lifestyle itself: reduce the number of anonymous sexual partners, know your partner and his sexual history, close the bathhouses, stop using poppers, stop having sex.

The discovery of a new sexually transmitted disease, one that destroyed the very mechanism that normally protected the body from diseases, posed a challenge to the future of homosexual sex itself. It led to a crisis not only about sex in general but also about the kinds of sex that gay men engaged in—fellatio, fisting, anal intercourse, casual sex with strangers and with multiple partners—with anal intercourse being one of the most efficient means of transmitting the disease. Anal sex has often been considered by many gay men one of the most valued aspects of their sexuality. "The rectum is a sexual organ," argued Joseph Sonnabend, a prominent HIV physician, "and it deserves the respect a penis gets and a vagina gets. Anal intercourse has been the central activity for gay men and some women for all of history. . . . We have to recognize what is hazardous, but at the same time, we shouldn't undermine an act that's important to celebrate."[1]

In the early days of the epidemic, many physicians and social critics—including gay activist and writer Larry Kramer—urged gay men to stop having sex.[2] But abstaining from sex completely was not considered a long-term option. Gay men developed safer sex guidelines that included an insistence on condom usage across a range of activities. These guidelines often felt like the unsexiest "to do" list:

- Step 1. Take out condom.
- Step 2. Take out lubrication.
- Step 3. Put a couple drops of lubrication on your penis.
- Step 4. Unwrap condom.
- Step 5. Lubricate his butthole.
- Step 6. Put condom on your penis.
- Step 7. Enter his anus.
- Step 8. Move back and forth until complete.
- Step 9. Remove condom carefully.
- Step 10. Tie off condom and throw in garbage (not the toilet!).

This "condom code" had nothing to do with desire or play or negotiation: it was designed to prevent the transmission of disease. Many critics believed that it failed to address the most significant factors underlying the epidemic: promiscuity and anal sex.

In large part, the widespread adoption of safer sex during the 1980s was in part motivated by fear. Many men, if not infected themselves, helped care for their dying friends and lovers, regularly attended memorials, and saw dying, wasted men walking the streets of gay communities in major cities. Community newspapers published dozens of obituaries in every issue, instilling not only fear about sex but also psychological wounds that damaged gay men's core identities. They were often left on their own to negotiate between the personal significance of the sex they engaged in and the community and public standards of "safer" sex.

In 1995, *New York Magazine* reported that "the return of vintage seventies promiscuity has sparked a small boom in theaters, dance clubs, bars, and a variety of other venues that have back rooms and private cubicles for sex."[3] Although many men who practice unprotected sex do so because they believe that condoms lessen the pleasure, some see their sexual activity as a form of resistance to "health" as a moral imperative, embodied in the belief that risk reduction is a rational norm. Unprotected sexual activity is, thus, one response to the historical trauma of HIV experienced by gay men: the health of gay men and their physical survival remain live issues.

For those who grew up in the HIV epidemic, the claim that they could "return to vintage seventies promiscuity" seems inaccurate: How could they return to a time they'd never experienced? Exploration is a necessary part of sexual identity, each generation finding its way through their bodies and sexualities. Sex in its many forms, then, is part of the journey, part of the exchange, part of the community.

Notes

1. Quoted in Gabriel Rotello, *Sexual Ecology: AIDS and the Destiny of Gay Men* (New York: Plume, 1997), 101.

2. The most prominent of these critics inside the gay male community is Larry Kramer, "1,112 and Counting," *New York Native*, March 14–27, 1983. See also his *Reports from the Holocaust: The Making of An AIDS Activist*, (New York: St. Martin's Press, 1989).

3. Craig Horowitze, "Has AIDS Won?," *New York Magazine*, February 20, 1995, 33.

4

Reluctant Objects

HIV Prevention and the Problem of Sexual Pleasure

KANE RACE

In treating pleasure ultimately as nothing other than an event, an event that happens, that happens, I would say, outside the subject, or at the limit of the subject, or between two subjects, in this some-thing that is neither of the body nor of the soul, neither outside nor inside—don't we have here, in trying to reflect a bit on this notion of pleasure, a means of avoiding the entire psychological and medical armature that was built into the traditional notion of desire?
—Michel Foucault, "The Gay Science"

The controversy over PrEP and gay sex speaks to how condoms have served to manage communal fears about sexual excess in the era of AIDS, providing not only a latex barrier but also symbolic reassurance that gay sex might in some way be made "safe." It is symbolic because, given its clinical efficacy, the characterization of PrEP use as "irresponsible" could make sense only in a world in which the problem that HIV prevention is supposed to address is not simply viral transmission but is also the moral danger attributed to gay sexual pleasure in general. From this perspective, PrEP commentary is reminiscent of "the comfortable fantasy that AIDS would spell the end of gay promiscuity, or perhaps gay sex altogether"—an observation Bersani originally made about the hygienic measures proposed in the intensely homophobic climate of the early epidemic.[1] It is not the first time that antiviral medications have provoked anxieties about the moral climate of gay sex. As early as 1997, Douglas Crimp observed that a pervasive and recurring theme in Andrew Sullivan's well-known essay "When Plagues End" was the "fear that these new drugs will give gay men the freedom to go back to their old promiscuous habits"—a point that appears as applicable to today's otherwise radically transformed present as it was persuasive then.[2]

PrEP: Initial Apprehensions

This chapter was first designed as a modest intervention into a situation in which science would render sexual encounters dumb. It began as a speculative exercise that attempted to make sense of gay men's initial reactions to PrEP. My argument emerged from a series of encounters and an overall impression—based on my participation in gay culture—of what I would characterize as a surprising state of disengagement with PrEP. PrEP takes the shape of a reluctant object: an object that may well make a tangible difference to people's lives, but whose promise is so threatening or confronting to enduring habits of getting by in this world that it provokes aversion, avoidance, and even condemnation and moralism. Thinking about gay men's initial engagement (or rather disengagement) with PrEP stands to tell us much about their self-understanding as subjects of risk in the present moment of the epidemic, providing insight into those circumstances in which one is led to turn away, to linger in a state of non-confrontation, to avoid recognizing oneself as a subject of risk.[3] The object of PrEP forces us to contend with what scares us—not only about risk but also about sex; for example, how the condom has operated in the citizenship arena both as a latex and a symbolic prophylactic against the apparently terrifying prospect of unbridled homosexuality. Approaching PrEP as a reluctant object—an object that, in its current enactment, has largely failed to engage its intended subjects—might serve as an occasion to rethink the space of the research encounter and to generate new research objects, subjects, and forms of relation.

Before proceeding further, some words of qualification are in order. By positioning PrEP as a "reluctant object," I do not mean to suggest that it is an unproblematic object or that concerns about it are unfounded. PrEP poses considerable challenges regarding its effective implementation, use, and resourcing, all of which require serious consideration. The issues of nonadherence, risk compensation, cost, access, unwanted toxicity, and the possible development of resistant viruses in the context of undetected seroconversion and suboptimal treatment (which is what PrEP would be in these circumstances) are real and must be addressed.[4] (The latter—suboptimal treatment—possibility vividly demonstrates how biomedical objects may be ontologically transformed in their encounter with other entities and practices.) But in this chapter, I bracket these concerns, because these are not the main ones I typically encountered when raising the issue of PrEP with HIV-negative sexual partners and friends in casual discussion. As of 2022, people outside the HIV sector had not even got that far in thinking about

PrEP, in my experience. Rather, my aim here is to understand the affective reaction with which news of PrEP is often greeted: a reaction of aversion—often powerful aversion and repudiation—among men who are otherwise familiar with and often have more or less sensible and considered approaches to the challenges of HIV prevention. Understanding these reactions may be useful for thinking through how health services and educators might present PrEP to relevant publics. It might also help frame HIV prevention as a matter of affective attachments and investments: that is, how people come to attach themselves to particular objects, practices, devices, positions, and identities in their attempts to avoid—or otherwise navigate—the possibility of HIV infection.

That is, the aim of this work is not to psychologize HIV-negative gay men, as though PrEP were an object that rational folks cannot but want. I object to those forms of psychological reasoning that take the latest health prescription as an opportunity to pathologize the noncompliant, and I would want to situate the range of reactions more sympathetically in their historical and practical contexts and generative potential. Instead, my hope in pursuing this topic is to contribute to a discussion about how gay men relate to HIV—especially in circumstances where their practices may be associated with risk. I want to question whether the model of the prudent, rational pre-calculative subject of risk that we customarily work with in the field adequately imagines how we enter into sex.[5]

This work is also motivated by the immense difficulty I have experienced as an HIV-positive man involved in the field not only in thinking about PrEP but also in trying to imagine how things must appear and be experienced by those with a different serostatus. Rather than interpret this difficulty as some sort of personal shortcoming, in this chapter I install it as a methodological starting point and default presumption inspired by work on interesting science: we do not know what is going on for other people and must presume not to know and be prepared to be surprised by our encounters.[6] In other words, my thinking emerges from my own initial reluctance to think about PrEP . . . and then a series of dumb questions and confronting encounters.

A Few Dumb Questions

I posted a link on my Facebook page in April 2012 to an article titled "A Game-Changer in the Fight against HIV," from the *Boston Globe*.[7] The article was a straightforward, well-written account that outlined the findings from PrEP trials and described the prophylactic as a promising strategy. Given how fed up we are thirty years on with the persistence of this epidemic and considering the widespread desire for an end to it, you would think that news like this would attract a little attention. But from among my bevvy of overtly gay Facebook friends, shown posing at gyms and parties and parades, only one person "liked" it. Even news about what I had for breakfast attracts more attention.

Now it would be foolish to draw any strict conclusions from this flimsy piece of "data," and there are a number of ways to interpret the findings. Perhaps it was the wrong time of day, or a newsfeed issue, or a problem with my recruitment strategy (my friends are very odd and unrepresentative, after all). Perhaps it indicates a case of information overload, or there were other more captivating things going on at the time. Difficult as this line of questioning is to disentangle from the narcissistic preoccupations of Facebook interaction more generally, these considerations can usefully be brought to any survey, online or otherwise. Data are always mediated by the sociotechnical arrangements that make them available to us, and it is good to get specific about these techniques and mediations. Ever the social researcher, I decided to consult with another expert in this particular medium and asked my boyfriend what this appalling response rate could be about. "Well, 'liking' it could be taken as an admission of wanting or having unsafe sex," he said, "something that people are reluctant to identify themselves with in public."

This interpretation is valuable and interesting, not because it is representative or definitive in any way but because it gives us partial insight into some of the conditions of articulation and silence around PrEP. Expressing a personal interest in PrEP means acknowledging to oneself and to others that one's practices are not as safe as they could or "ought" to be. This observation could help us begin to understand the apparent absence of public expressions of demand for PrEP to date—an issue that has flummoxed many clinical researchers in the area. But it also opens a broader series of considerations. Engaging personally with PrEP involves confronting oneself not only as a subject of risk but also as a subject of illicit or socially unsanctioned sex.

This PrEP exchange on social media occurred after sex with a 25-year-old HIV-negative man at his home. We had used condoms, which were conveniently at hand: the guy was clearly well versed in the practices of arranging safe, casual sex. After sex we got into a discussion about our interests and work, and I raised the topic of PrEP. The topic needed some explanation. While he was educated, seemed to be savvy about HIV prevention, and had a vague sense of having heard about something along these lines, he was unclear of the details or of what the treatment might be like. After my explanation, he grew quite animated and disturbed: I was surprised at how upset he became. He could not understand why people could not just use condoms. On further discussion it emerged that he had previously been in a one- or two-year relationship with an HIV-positive man. He had managed to sustain condom use even in these challenging circumstances, so he believed condoms should be a sufficient prevention strategy.

How can we understand this objection to PrEP and its relation to an attachment to condoms? This is where considerations of affect and habituation are useful, and I am inclined to theorize condoms along these lines as a difficult but nonetheless optimistic attachment. Condom use is a hard-wrought attachment—a carefully habituated practice—that incorporates the condom into an affectively charged and potentially disorganizing scene of intensity. Despite the difficulty of this attachment and the conditions that militate against it, many gay men have managed to install condom use as a habitual and ongoing practice.

I am interested in the sense in which this habituation might be considered to have staved off the unbearable immediacy of the threat of HIV/AIDS. Of interest here are the processes through which condom use is transformed from a decisional event into a practice—that is, a matter of habit. It might be presumed that consistent condom use is an instance of effective interpellation into risk discourse. After all, is this not precisely what HIV educators want gay men to do? In becoming used habitually, the condom acquires a form that provides a measure of freedom beyond immediacy, putting off the unsustainable "decisionism of a life lived minute to minute"—that is, in a crisis mentality.[8] One thing that condoms have been good for, in other words, is to enable one to avoid thinking too much—and too intimately—about what at some level is unthinkable: the threat of HIV/AIDS.[9] If condoms have functioned as a way to preserve a mode of ordinariness in a situation of unendurable and ongoing crisis, then this would overturn our usual assumptions about the decisionality of safe sex. When in the mode of consistency, we do not decide to use condoms: rather, they are used habitually, unthinkingly, and doing so operates as a source of comfort. The condom habit may in this sense be a way to exempt oneself from a repeated and traumatic interpellation by risk discourse. From this perspective, it operates as a habitual way to avoid the question. Of course, there are other mechanisms for doing this, but the condom is perhaps least problematic and also happens to have some beneficial side effects, such as preventing HIV transmission! Consider the assumption, typical among some peers, that we are not the intended recipients of these irritating, never-ending safe sex messages and campaigns; those other evil barebackers/young gay men/scene queens/sex addicts (fill in the appropriate "other") are.

In the context of this attachment to condoms—which is at once often difficult and optimistic—and the emotional energy and investment it involves, PrEP is likely to materialize as both a threatening proposition and a challenging interference.[10] What it threatens is not simply the subject's preferences or convictions with regard to HIV prevention but the sense of continuity provided by habituated adherence to a particular formal investment in the cluster of promises that is encapsulated in more established preventive objects. From this perspective, the moralism that surrounds PrEP might be understood as a way to counter the threat that a different logic—a different package for delivering on this cluster of promises—poses to this hard-wrought and strenuously maintained attachment.

This is a relevant consideration, I think, for proponents of PrEP, who must find ways to anticipate and respond to this sort of resistance. It is analogous to the resistance first encountered in discussions of "negotiated safety" that posed a similar sort of threat to investments in the formal structure of safe sex.[11] "Negotiated safety" was the formulation of Australian social researchers and educators who noticed that some gay men were dispensing with condoms with regular partners of the same HIV status while using them in more casual sexual contexts outside the relationship. Researchers saw that this practice could operate as a form of HIV prevention. Coined at a time of immense investment in the condom as the primary guarantor of safety, the concept of negotiated safety sparked immense controversy internationally. As it proliferated in scientific circles and community discourse, the controversy revealed how powerfully an object such as the condom can become stabilized as a placeholder for the investment of anxious energies, as well as what happens when the continuity of its form is brought into question. One insight that can be drawn from this episode is the challenge implicit in affirming some people's commitment to consistent condom use while presenting and describing PrEP to those who may need or serve to benefit from it. Although some proponents insist that PrEP is not a replacement for condoms but rather a supplement, I do not think that this insistence is realistic. It fails to anticipate how PrEP materializes in practical terms, not only as an option but also as a substitute—and, for some, a source of interference. What it interferes with is the self-evidence of those attachments and associations that have constituted one of the most basic and enduring ontologies of HIV prevention for many gay men, specifically those embodied, formalized, and authorized in the principle of "safe sex."

To help us think further about this question of effectively targeting and articulating PrEP among those who most stand to benefit from it, my next anecdote raises more questions about how people come to recognize themselves as subjects of risk and possible candidates for PrEP. This encounter involved a discussion over dinner with an HIV-negative friend, a thoughtful, intelligent, and frank Sydney resident about my age. We had engaged in discussions before about different experiences of serostatus and sex. Again, I was surprised to find that he had never heard about, or considered, the issue of PrEP. His initial response, when I described it, was marked trepidation and surprise. It struck him as a "brave new world" proposition that might open the gates to unbridled sex. Not that there is anything prudish or conservative about my friend—quite the contrary, as it happens. But when I asked for clarification in a later communication, he wrote ruefully, "I can imagine people stocking up on it pre-Mardi Gras and then behaving like cars at a service station all weekend . . . 'Fill er up!'"—before he went on to qualify the associations as he saw them, "but I also meant in the novel's sense of strange Sci-Fi medicine and how that affects culture." On this occasion, PrEP raised the specter of limitless sex and fears of a technologically transformed world—propositions that seem both scary and thrilling and, for this reason, can prompt defenses.

One thing that perplexed my friend most about PrEP was the temporal relation to risk that it seemed to represent. Despite—or perhaps because of—all the efforts to enlist us as prudent and pre-calculative subjects of health, we are in the habit of accounting for sexual risk—taking after the event, as he went on to observe. The representation implicit in PrEP of risk as premeditated is at once more confronting and a different way to identify the self in the vicinity of risk, not to mention account for that relation. It relies on the sense of a predictive and intentional subject whose propensity to err is fully present and apprehensible to that subject in advance. This led to a search for comparisons, during which I suggested the contraceptive pill. But my friend rejected the analogy on the grounds that a pregnancy is terminable, whereas HIV is not—or "not yet." (I am not as convinced about this distinction myself, because an unwanted pregnancy may sometimes pose a similar crisis of self-viability for women. The similarities and differences between PrEP, the contraceptive pill, and their historical reception certainly deserve further consideration.) This line of conversation led into a discussion of his own sexual and risk practices, in which he divulged that he had been taking more risks in the recent past, that it had been difficult to maintain condom use, and that he had surprised even himself with the risks he had been prepared to consider in recent memory. Situations that might just a year ago have seemed to him unthinkably risky were now ones in which he found himself tempted to participate.

There is a lot that could be said about this conversation, and in many ways, it corresponds with other recent discussions I have had with sexually active gay friends that seem to lend some urgency to the search for new HIV prevention strategies, including PrEP. But for this investigation, the main point I want to make is that, even though on reflection my friend was concerned about risk and about his own inclination to take risks (which he perceived as increasing), PrEP was still encountered as a challenging proposition that he experienced some difficulty engaging. What can we make of this difficulty? What is going on here, and what can we draw from this encounter?

The Paradox of the Planned Slipup

I believe that, from a certain perspective, at this point in the epidemic PrEP emerges as an enigmatic object: the paradox of a planned slipup. It asks us to preempt a possibility that we have become accustomed to accounting for mainly after the event or as an afterthought. As a proposition, PrEP asks HIV-negative men not only to acknowledge but also take systematic, prescribed, coordinated, and involved action against a risk that one may not be inclined to acknowledge so readily. Or a risk that one may acknowledge at some level but that is rationalized as not much of a risk—or as something that happens spontaneously, irregularly, or in the heat of the moment—perhaps in a bid to protect oneself from confronting the self-interpretation that would consist in understanding one's risk practice as becoming habitual.[12]

It is interesting to contrast this particular orientation to risk with the figure of the barebacker, whose self-identification could be interpreted paradoxically as an ideal instance of interpellation into contemporary risk discourse. The term "barebacking" emerged in the late 1990s and was quickly defined in the scientific and popular literature alike as the apparently new phenomenon of "intentional unsafe sex"—although some commentators were quick to question the universality of this descriptor. Intentionality does not even begin to describe the full range of relations to unprotected sex, as Barry Adam pointed out in an early article on the topic.[13] Nevertheless, the term inspired popular identification with a speed and force that revealed the poverty of dominant modes of accounting for sexual risk practices, which at their base seem always to require and impute an intentional subject who is free to exercise any choice he or she pleases in any given circumstance. Given this history, the self-identified barebacker might be considered the exemplary subject of neoliberal risk discourse.[14] His willingness to "own" risk in the mode of foresight and intentionality can be taken to situate him quite firmly in the neighborhood of PrEP's presumed address.

By contrast, the reluctant subject does not locate himself at this address and loiters in a state of nonconfrontation with regard to risk. In a curious way, then, PrEP emerges as the counterfigure of the conundrum that informs some gay men's use of recreational substances to negotiate the pressures of the prevention discourse that I described in *Pleasure Consuming Medicine* as "Exceptional Sex."[15] On such occasions, risk takes on the structure of the exception, in a manner that is at once pre-calculated but disavowed, planned for but not fully acknowledged. Relying on what the popular concept of disinhibition makes available by way of explanations for disapproved behavior, the subject "gives himself a chance to swoon" and escape the pressure of the condom imperative.[16] The paradox here is that this notion of disinhibition is a discourse that is largely apprehended in advance. Thus, drug use serves as a way to avoid the charge of intentionality.

By comparison, PrEP asks HIV-negative men to confront the structure of exception head-on: to identify themselves as subjects of risk in the mode of pre-calculation and intentionality. Perhaps, then, PrEP is such a reluctant object partly because it makes explicit something that is difficult to be explicit about from within one of the common orientations to sex and risk among gay men today: the desire to position risk as an exception rather than a tendency, a "straying afield of oneself" rather than something as coherent or culpable as a habit or a precalculated decision.

As I said in the beginning of the chapter, these thoughts are necessarily speculative, partial, and incomplete. I see this work as a contribution to the body of literature that turns to sex and pleasure as modes of relationality and encounter that query the models of proper personhood idealized in the notion of the sovereign, prudent, preemptive, intentional subject who is presumed to be always capable of performing risk-benefit calculations in advance.[17] The affective responses I described in this chapter should not be seen as essential psychological reactions that precede PrEP and that determine how we respond to it once and forevermore but as prehensions: that is, variable ways to grasp things that are bound up in the actualization of events.[18] Apprehensions of PrEP will change as PrEP enters into various forms of circulation, and it is difficult to predict just what will take place and how. It will depend, in part, on how sex, risk, and prevention are scientifically, discursively, and practically enacted by science and other institutional practices; hence, my attention to research methods. A guiding premise of this chapter is that subjects emerge in relation with specific objects and the manner of their creation: subjects and objects are coproduced. This marks out a more active role for research practices than might usually be assumed. For whatever else it is, PrEP is an event: "All those who are touched by an event define and are defined by it"; they become part of the event's effects.[19] By engaging relations between risk, sex, and prevention science, this chapter has sought to participate in this process of eventuation.

One question I hope to develop in future work is what to make of such refusals of prevention and care, as I describe them here. This is a matter whose significance is prompted by the recent experience of PrEP but extends well beyond it, because there are broader questions about the reluctance of marginalized subjects to access care that acquire particular significance in the biomedical prevention context. These questions are not simply psychological but also implicate much wider socio-material arrangements and attachments: the political production of multiple worlds.[20] That is, although the line of inquiry I develop in this chapter might seem like just another set of reasons to put PrEP into the "too hard" basket, on the contrary I believe it represents an opportunity to do the sort of thinking that is needed to address subjects of risk, pleasure, sexuality, and HIV in their present complexity. This is a methodological and not simply a conceptual challenge, as I have insisted throughout. I have been testing the value of engaging more openly and attentively in intimate and unsettling encounters and the way they move our thinking . . . from science to the sex that eventuates.

Notes

I am grateful to the Canadian Social Research Centre in HIV Prevention and the Center for the Study of Sexualities at National Central University Taiwan for the opportunities they provided to present and discuss this research. I would like to thank Mike Michael, Marsha Rosengarten, Heather Love, Meaghan Morris, Elspeth Probyn, Hans Huang, Susan Kippax, Niamh Stephenson, Robert Grant, Trevor Hoppe, Judith Auerbach, Dean Murphy, Mathieu Trachman, Jeff McConnell, Nick Perrett, Ariel Fefer, and Adrian Kerr for encouraging conversations that helped me develop this article, as well as two anonymous peer reviewers from GLQ whose criticisms prompted me to sharpen its argument. Michel Foucault, "The Gay Science," *Critical Inquiry* 37, no. 3 (Spring 2011): 385–403.

1. Leo Bersani, "Is the Rectum a Grave?" in *AIDS: Cultural Analysis, Cultural Activism*, ed. Douglas Crimp (Cambridge, MA: MIT Press, 1988), 106.

2. Douglas Crimp, *Melancholia and Moralism: Essays on AIDS and Queer Politics* (Cambridge, MA: MIT Press, 2004) 287. Interestingly, Andrew Sullivan recently took Larry Kramer to task in a blog post that seems to indicate a partial shift in Sullivan's apprehension of sexual practice in the post-AIDS context.

3. If, for Althusser, interpellation describes the "hey you!" moment when individuals recognize themselves as subjects of official discourse, one way to frame this section might be as an inquiry into the conditions of uninterpellation; see his *Essays on Ideology* (New York: Verso, 1970). But this term brings with it all the baggage of "ideological state apparatuses," a dense and determining set of structures (both theoretically and ontologically) that one may well wish to avoid for this reason. Luckily, some

equally viable ways to frame this problem can be drawn from science studies, where the case has been made for treating recalcitrant figures and their ontological attachments seriously, even engaging the "idiot" as a productive occasion for rethinking the organizing principles of entrenched paradigms of knowledge and practice. See Michel Callon and Vololona Rebehariosa, "Gino's Lesson on Humanity: Generics, Mutual Entanglements, and the Sociologist's Role," *Economy and Society* 33, no. 1 (2004): 1–24; and Mike Michael, "What Are We Busy Doing?" Engaging the Idiot," *Science, Technology, and Human Values* 37, no. 5 (2011) 528–554.

4. See generally, Mark Wainberg, "Pre-Exposure Prophylaxis against HIV: Pros and Cons," *Retrovirology* 9, suppl. 1 (2012): 16.

5. For a classic elaboration of this model of the subject, see Nikolas Rose, *Inventing Our Selves* (Cambridge: Cambridge University Press, 1998), 150–168.

6. Bruno Latour, "How to Talk about the Body: The Normative Dimension of Science Studies," *Body and Society* 10, nos. 2–3 (2004): 205–229; and Isabelle Stengers, *Power and Invention: Situating Science* (Minneapolis: University of Minnesota Press, 1997), as discussed earlier.

7. Sean Cahill, "A Game-Changer in the Fight against HIV," *Boston Globe*, March 26, 2012.

8. Lauren Berlant, *Cruel Optimism* (Durham, NC: Duke University Press, 2011), 63.

9. In a phrase that could aptly describe the outbreak of AIDS and its initial apprehension as a community crisis, Berlant focuses our attention on the "drama of adjustment to a pervasive atmosphere of unexpected precarity." In these circumstances, according to Berlant, people desperately seek out a habit or a form that might help preserve the energy it would take to live in a heightened state of unbearable immediacy. Adjusting to living with HIV can be described from this perspective as a question of how we "learn to submit to the passivity and the activity of

feeling forced to take on living as a practice, on the way to the deliberate mode becoming a habit, a comfortable gestural rhythm." Berlant, *Cruel Optimism*, 62.

10. The term *interference* is used by science studies scholars such as Annemarie Mol and John Law to refer to the threat posed by one ontology to another (or multiple others) in the context of multiplicity. For these scholars, the strength and robustness of a particular ontology are always dependent on the various networks, associations, attachments, and practices that hold it in place as a stable and enduring reality. Because other networks, associations attachments, and practices always coexist, sometimes in tension, ontologies are said to "interfere with" one another. But this interference may be more or less antagonistic, serious, consequential, or endurable because of circumstances such as proximity or the relative availability of the tension to be ushered into some sort of practical or negotiated coexistence. See generally Annemarie Mol, *The Body Multiple: Ontology in Medical Practice* (Durham, NC: Duke University Press, 2003); and John Law, *After Method: Mess in Social Science Research* (London: Routledge, 2004).

11. For an account, see Kane Race, "The Difference Practice Makes: Evidence, Articulation, and Affect in HIV Prevention," *AIDS Education and Prevention: An Interdisciplinary Journal* 26, no. 3 (2014): 256–266.

12. Another HIV-negative friend in the same age group described PrEP to me in similar terms as "wearing a bullet-proof vest across the road." As a comment on forms of precautionary behavior, this analogy constructs PrEP in terms of overkill and as a course of action that is not well fit to the risks at hand. The person who used this analogy has unprotected casual sex regularly within what he regards as "tried and true" risk assumptions and parameters.

13. Barry Adam, "Constructing the Neoliberal Sexual Actor: Responsibility and Care of the Self in the Discourse of

Barebackers," *Culture, Health and Sexuality* 7, no. 4 (2005): 333–346.

14. Adam, "Constructing the Neoliberal Sexual Actor."

15. Kane Race, *Pleasure Consuming Medicine: The Queer Politics of Drugs* (Durham, NC: Duke University Press, 2009) 164–190.

16. Michael Warner describes this as "the poppers effect" in *The Trouble with Normal: Sex, Politics, and the Ethics of Queer Life* (New York: Free Press, 1999), 213.

17. See Judith Butler, *Giving an Account of Oneself* (New York: Fordham University Press, 2005). On the logic of preemption as a mode of neoliberal governmentality, see Melinda Cooper, "Pre-Empting Emergence: The Biological Turn in the War on Terror," *Theory, Culture and Society* 23, no. 4 (2006): 113–134; Brian Massumi, "Potential Politics and the Primacy of Pre-Emption," *Theory and Event* 10, no. 2 (2007): 1–34.

18. Alfred North Whitehead, *Process and Reality, An Essay on Cosmology*, rev. ed. (1978; repr. New York: Free Press, 1929).

19. Mariam Fraser, "Fact, Ethics and Event," in *Deleuzian Intersections: Science, Technology, Anthropology*, ed. Casper Jensen and Kjetil Rodje (New York: Berghahn Books, 2013), 65.

20. Callon and Rebeharisoa, "Gino's Lesson," and Mol, *Body Multiple*.

5

Learning How to Fuck on PrEP

NIC FLORES

Ideally, fucking should be fun, stress-free, and pleasurable for everyone involved. When we consider the contemporary arrangements and energies around sex, and bareback fucking in particular, we notice that something is happening. In dominant modes of medical and public health discourses, sex is still unwittingly relegated to the side of either respectability or promiscuity. Both sides illuminate how the various boundaries around fucking—how it is felt, who is doing it, and what pleasures are derived from it—reveal it as a socially dynamic and emergent activity. Keeping this in mind, my interest here is in the lessons to be learned and unlearned about how we come to fuck while on PrEP in the world today.

The title of my chapter, "Learning How to Fuck on PrEP," enters the ongoing conversations about the implementation and uptake of the biomedical intervention known as pre-exposure prophylaxis (PrEP) among Black and Brown communities in the United States. Introduced to the U.S. market in 2012, the once-a-day pill is used alongside antiretroviral (ARV) medications to reduce viral suppression and to curb transmission rates among HIV-negative people.[1] This chapter draws from my fieldwork conducted between 2016 and 2018, focusing on one ethnographic anecdote. Far from presenting PrEP as an uncritical, linear point of progress in the traumatic history of the virus, I understand the pill and its effects as a continuity of the sexual racism and structural vulnerability that constitute the virus.[2]

Getting and Giving a PrEP Education

"His face looked so confused when I explained how PrEP worked," stated Elias, a late twenty-something, self-identified "Latinx cis-male" living in central Ohio.[3] As he described this scene with an anonymous sexual partner he met through a phone dating application, he continued, "I mean, I had to tell him that we didn't need to use a condom since I was on [PrEP] and that it prevented HIV. Even though he was confused and initially reluctant, we eventually fucked raw. It was hot and worth that brief explanation."[4] On reflecting further, Elias concluded, "Honestly, it was kind of strange that I had to explain this to a white guy—I don't normally hook up with white dudes. I feel like [PrEP] is a thing that white gays know more about. At least, that's been my experience."[5] After we wrapped up the interview, I reflected on the broader systemic implications and the multiple scales through which this encounter was conditioned and experienced: the historical precedence of the virus within and among minoritized communities, (mis)understandings about HIV prevention, contemporary medical breakthroughs, bareback sex, and communication about how encounters are negotiated in intimate spaces in real time.

Questions emerged: How did Elias—and others—come to their understandings about bareback sex once on PrEP? In what ways do our social positions and situatedness inform how we communicate about PrEP to sex partners and then engage in sex acts? What types of relations are being forged through the use of biomedical interventions like PrEP? And, keeping the previous question in mind, what types of social relations are eclipsed through bareback pleasure seeking among racially sexualized subjects?

This type of encounter—a "quick fuck" with an educational moment—was not Elias's first foray into clarifying PrEP's significance to his casual partners. Indeed, others I interviewed similarly described its newfound role in their lives and the chance to experience condomless sex mostly carefree. The terms of his meeting, his recollection, and his translation of the scene to me seemed, at first, aligned with others' stories about the various scales of understanding themselves on PrEP. At the time of our interview (2017) there was an increase in educational information about PrEP, with much of it coming to people via social media. In this encounter, Elias was in the position not only of knower (explaining how PrEP works) but also of knowledge producer through the sex act. Elias, like others whom I interviewed about their experiences on PrEP, would take on the simultaneous role of sex educator and pleasure seeker.

Black and Brown gay and queer men's sexual encounters and high-risk sex are increasingly the main topics of concern in HIV prevention in both public health discourses and popular culture. Many who laud its arrival claim that PrEP offers chances to explore sexual interests, intimacies, and pleasures through sexual acts that have accrued forbidden and taboo meanings since the 1980s. However, the double-edged sword of the virus's disproportionate impact on Black and Brown communities reveals the contradictions within these logics and discourses. On the one hand, the body of information about gay sex unwittingly vilifies certain sexual acts like bareback sex and, by extension, those who choose to engage in them. On the other hand, those bodies that are disproportionately higher in rates of transmission fall along racial, ethnic, and class lines. The epidemiological knowledges produced about and around HIV's disproportionate impact among Black and Brown communities unwittingly castigate sexual acts deemed high risk without fuller understandings of the structural complexities at play, including accessibility, health care coverage, personal dispositions about the medical field, and mistrust.

Unlearning PrEP's Whiteness

Performance studies scholar Peggy Phelan writes that the "power of the 'unseen' community lies in its ability to cohere outside the system of observation which seeks to patrol it."[6] Inversely, it is precisely through the seen and knowable that Black and Brown PrEP users are able to mark whiteness's presence as a social force in their worlds. Whiteness is not only social context and an unmarked common but also a social logic that both produces and substantiates unequal social relations, a discourse made material through PrEP's unequal distribution and consumption by certain racialized bodies. Don't believe me? Ask your friends who is and is not on PrEP. This process of racialization that followed PrEP's uptake accentuates what George Lipsitz refers to as the "possessive investment in whiteness." For Lipsitz, social life is figured as "the sum total of conscious and deliberative individual activities," which cloaks "racist" activity as "individual manifestations of personal prejudice and hostility."[7] By maintaining social arrangements in which individuals and their activities remain the locus of political activity, "systemic, collective, and coordinated group behavior consequently drops of out of sight," argues Lipsitz [8] It's much easier to blame an individual for being racist than to consider the systems, structures, and institutions that affect how and why people operate in white supremacist orders, knowingly or not. The weight placed on individuality reifies, by both validating openly and hiding in plain sight, an investment in whiteness as a social, structural, and health-related advantage. If Phelan's theorization draws our attention to that which is unseen and unmarked, then Lipsitz forces us to consider how whiteness attaches to certain bodies as a way to configure social spaces, especially HIV prevention work, by "giving people from different races vastly different life chances."[9]

From Unlearning to Relearning to Healing

The process of learning is equally about unlearning and then relearning. In his seminal essay, "How to Have Promiscuity in an Epidemic," the late Douglas Crimp writes, "Our promiscuity taught us many things, not only about the pleasures of sex, but about the great multiplicity of those pleasures."[10] Buried within Crimp's forceful articulations and arguments concerning the limitations of the earlier "gays rights movement" are provocations and demands for those of us committed to justice to do better. In short, to learn, unlearn, and relearn.

I shared Elias's interview about educating his sexual partner about PrEP and the implications it had on his encounter to show how the lessons and fucking among Black and Brown communities differ from those of their white counterparts. His encounter and my brief analysis are not meant to stand in as hard evidence of what we can fully understand as the messiness of sex today. Rather, I share his encounter to illuminate the assumptive logics and lessons about fucking and, in particular, about the fucking we think we're having. For better or worse, learning how to fuck on PrEP means facing shame, stigma, and sexual racism within gay cis-male communities and having the audacity to name it and change it. Learning, in many unexpected and unanticipated ways, is also about unlearning and, we hope, healing.

PrEP has not only enabled certain forms of bodily arrangements through sexual acts but has also offered new possibilities for shared intimacy and pleasure across difference. Now is the time to pause, reflect, and interrogate the transformations that HIV prevention and sex education have undergone. Above all else, it is the time to heal as we continue to learn how to fuck on PrEP.

Notes

1. Robert M. Grant, Javier R. Lama, Peter L. Anderson, Vanessa McMahan, Albert Y. Liu, Lorena Vargas, Pedro Goicochea, Martín Casapía, et al., "Preexposure Chemoprophylaxis for HIV Prevention in Men Who Have Sex with Men," *New England Journal of Medicine* 363, no. 27 (2010): 2587–2599. doi:10.1056/NEJMoa1011205.

2. I draw on Marlon M. Bailey's use of the term "structural vulnerability" to describe health disparities faced by and particular to gay Black men. I extend and include the particularities of Latinx men, too, who share similarities but are not reducible to them. Additionally, Sonja Mackenzie's theorizations around "structural intimacies" among Black people living with HIV inform my understandings. See Marlon M. Bailey, "Black Gay (Raw) Sex," in *No Tea, No Shade: New Writings in Black Queer Studies*, ed. E. Patrick Johnson (Durham: Duke University Press, 2016), 239–261; Sonja Mackenzie, *Structural Intimacies: Sexual Stories in the Black AIDS Epidemic* (New Brunswick: Rutgers University Press, 2013).

3. I use a pseudonym to protect the privacy and maintain confidentiality of my interlocuters.

4. Interview with author.

5. Interview with author.

6. Peggy Phelan, *Unmarked: The Politics of Performance* (London: Routledge, 1993), 97.

7. George Lipsitz, *The Possessive Investment in Whiteness: How White People Profit from Identity Politics* (Philadelphia: Temple University Press, 1998), 20.

8. Lipsitz, *The Possessive Investment*, 20.

9. Lipsitz, *The Possessive Investment*, 20.

10. Douglas Crimp, "How to Have Promiscuity in an Epidemic," *October* 43 (1987): 253. doi:10.2307/3397576.

6

Gay Sex Is Our Superpower

ALEX GARNER

Love wins, yet gay sex continues to be criminalized. As the mantra of "Love Wins" has taken hold, it has allowed our movements for liberation and equality to fall victim to some archaic notion of romantic love. This idealized notion of love among gays gives us legitimacy and respectability. It allows our heterosexual allies to see our noble quest for love as just like theirs. After all, love is love is love is love. Love lifts us up where we belong, and all you need is love. But what everyone seems to have overlooked is that we are not talking about love. We are not fighting for the right to love. What we are talking about is sex: the ability for two people of the same gender to engage in sexual activity. This is, and always has been, the root of our movement, and it remains our most underutilized power.

Gay sex is criminalized in nearly seventy countries around the world. Gay men continue to be arrested, tortured, imprisoned, and, in some cases, killed, all for the crime of having gay sex. In Indonesia, gay men are arrested and publicly tortured.[1] In Chechnya, gay men are imprisoned in internment camps and tortured.[2] In Iran, gay men are murdered in "honor killings" by loving family members.[3] Yet it seems as if every day we are reminded that love wins. If this is what winning looks like, then how do we possibly understand what it means to lose—our dignity, our rights, and our lives?

Gay marriage has come to epitomize the triumph of love. Heterosexual allies attend the celebrations as if they are the social events of the season. They spend too much on that Cuisinart juicer, but it's ok, it's a celebration of love. They sit there and watch the grooms in their matching Gucci suits, and they imagine them picking out the ideal china pattern to match the creamy white cabinetry in their luxuriously designed Santa Barbara kitchen.

But when the time comes for the grooms to kiss, it's a momentary reminder of the sex between the two men. These heterosexual guests can't bring themselves to imagine one smartly dressed groom balls deep in the other groom, bent over the marble countertop as the china crashes to the floor. The idealized heterosexual ally recoils, and we counter by stepping back. We've argued that sex is private: it's something that happens behind closed doors, and it shouldn't matter what we do in the bedroom. But it does matter. It has always mattered. And until 2003 it was still constitutional in the United States to arrest gay men for what we did in the privacy of our bedrooms.[4]

It's understandable that love came to exemplify the LGBT movement. It was perfect timing. The AIDS crisis forced us to talk openly about the sex we were having because HIV and the abject failure of our government were killing us. But once antiretrovirals transformed the epidemic and kept people alive, the community seized the opportunity of the post-AIDS era, pushed sex into the private realm, and rebranded our movement as a cause for love.

The new era of "love is love" began. Gay men hosted boozy brunches where they could debate and defend choosing the wedding colors of blush and bashful. Frenzied finances made possible elaborate flash mob proposals in hopes of going viral on social media. And homophones could find shelter by attending the gay wedding of a random acquaintance.

All the while, gay sex lost, because gay men around the world continued to be persecuted for having sex with one another. But all was not lost. In the midst of criminalization, gay sex persisted. In fact, it always has. This is the single greatest testament to our strength and perseverance. Gay men continue to have sex.

For decades gay men have risked everything for sex. We've risked arrest; violence; loss of family, home, and employment; disease; and even death. Not because we are stupid or reckless but because gay sex has value and meaning. We've had to learn to navigate corrupt police, violent homophobes, and opportunistic extortionists because that sexual connection of pleasure, passion, and intimacy is worth everything. It's our one amazing unifying experience.

The centering of love in our movement wasn't just deeply misguided but it also completely overlooked and underestimated our greatest strength—gay sex. Gay sex is our superpower. We've endured devastating losses, and we are still able to come together and find a sexual connection. These social bonds fulfill us and allow us to foster community. Our sex is profoundly political because we navigate those most intensely hostile environments, yet we determine what we will do with our own bodies to pursue pleasure. The immense power behind that is nearly impossible to describe.

Our superpower is demonstrated all around us. Sometimes it is easy to identify, and other times we have had to look more closely. Lil Nas X is currently one of the most prominent demonstrators of the power of gay sex. He is a gay Black man who is audacious, unashamed, and unapologetically sexual, and he's winning the argument by embracing gay sex.[5] He is showing us all how it can be done on a global stage. Meanwhile everyday superheroes walk among us. The young gay guy in Cairo who uses an app for a hookup knowing there is a chance he could be arrested by the police. The gay man in Mexico who is openly HIV-positive and sexual in the face of violent threats. The gay guy in Jakarta who visits a gay sauna knowing it's possible the place could be raided by the police.

Gay sex may have moved from the center of our movement, but it is still central to our everyday lives. It's something of immeasurable pleasure and power, and we can still decide to use it to resist heteronormative structures and transform our lives and the world around us.

Notes

1. See https://www.reuters.com/article/us-indonesia-caning /indonesias-aceh-province-publicly-canes-two-gay-men -idUSKBN29Y1YP.

2. See https://youtu.be/_2KMm49B6pE.

3. See https://www.nbcnews.com/feature/nbc-out/gay-iranian -man-dead-alleged-honor-killing-rights-group-says-n1266995.

4. See https://www.lambdalegal.org/in-court/cases/lawrence-v -texas.

5. See https://www.bbc.com/culture/article/20210708-pops-gay -sexual-revolution.

Perspective

Pharma

What does it mean to have a body regulated by pills and liquids? There are supplements and medications for nearly every possible condition or function. We are barraged with messages in health care and in the media that we need to do something about ourselves, whether it's to get more sleep, to purge toxins, to gain weight or—more likely—to lose it. What does it mean to be targeted by giant pharmaceutical industries through advertisements, websites, advice from clinicians, and other education efforts? Gay men are subjects and objects in this pharmacological turn, as various technologies become part of the choices and behaviors associated with sex.

PrEP is not the first pharmaceutical product to have a potentially significant impact on sexual behavior. Treatments for syphilis, gonorrhea, and chlamydia (the 1940s); the oral contraceptive pill (the 1950 and 60s); and pills for male erectile dysfunction (Viagra, Cialis, Levitra, etc., in the 1990s) all preceded PrEP (introduced in the 2010s). In every case, debates ensued about their potential to encourage increased sexual or risky activity; that is, promiscuity. Few of those debates offered any realistic assessments of what eventually happened. The final outcome in these developments depends on the balance between the pharmaceutical technology owned by global corporations and what degree of control individuals have over their sexual behavior.

The contraceptive pill, as opposed to the condom, offered a biochemical technique to break the link between heterosexual sex and procreation. It was approved by the FDA in 1960. Advocates promoted the pill as preventing unwanted pregnancies, enabling happier marriages, and helping control explosive population growth; its opponents warned that it would encourage women, especially unmarried women, to engage in promiscuous sex. Some observers believed that the contraceptive pill caused the sexual revolution of the 1960s and 70s. But in fact, the pill had very different effects. One of its most significant effects was that giving married women more control over the timing of their pregnancies allowed them to enter the labor market in greater numbers than ever before.[1]

Viagra, the first pill for erectile dysfunction—or what used to be called "impotence"—was discovered by accident. Researchers at Pfizer found that erections were a side effect of a relatively ineffective drug they were developing for hypertension and angina pectoris (a form of heart disease). When they decided to repackage it and market it as a treatment for impotence, Pfizer was initially reluctant to advertise it for fear that it would be labeled as a "sex drug."[2] Originally it was marketed to older men (fifties+), but in recent years it has been marketed to much younger men in their thirties and forties.

Erectile dysfunction medications became pivotal in the use of recreational drugs and sex. Viagra and its ilk countered some drugs—such as crystal methamphetamine, cocaine, and alcohol—that can have a deadening effect on erections. They altered how and when sex with recreational drugs could occur. The party scene became an acceptable option for people who associated erections with sex.

Pre-exposure prophylaxis (PrEP), an antiretroviral, was developed for people who are HIV-negative to reduce their vulnerability to HIV acquisition; it became available in the United States in 2012. It is not only very expensive (thus limiting its availability to those with high incomes or health insurance) but also opposed by those who believed that it would encourage risky sexual behavior. PrEP does successfully reduce the rate of HIV transmission but is unable to prevent other sexually transmitted infections (STIs). The condom is still the only means to prevent many STIs. Thus, in some areas HIV transmissions have declined while the rates of STIs have increased.

In the case of STIs, the contraceptive pill, and PrEP, the technology being superseded is the condom. These developments are part of what trans theorist Paul Preciado has called the "sex-gender industrial complex," the emergence of a pharmaceutical apparatus based on a biochemical technology. The same period of the 1960s to 2010s also saw the development of biochemical and medical means for the production and modification of gender and sexual subjectivities.[3]

Notes

1. Elaine Tyler May, *American and the Pill: A History of Promise, Peril and Liberation* (New York: Basic Books, 2010).

2. Janice M. Irvine, "Selling Viagra," *Contexts* 5, no. 2 (2006): 39–44; Kyle MacNeill, "The Story of Viagra: The Little Blue Pill that Changed Sex Forever," *Vice*, March 29, 2018.

3. Paul Preciado, *Testo Junkie: Sex, Drugs and Biopolitics in the Pharmacopornographic Era* (New York: Feminist Press, 2013), 25–28.

7

"Heard about It Before, but Don't Know Where to Get It"

A Black Gay Man's Journey to Securing PrEP

DEION SCOTT HAWKINS

As our nation continues to grapple with HIV, it is important to acknowledge the vast strides that have been made in HIV advocacy. From enhancing access to care to reconceptualizing an HIV diagnosis as a chronic ailment as opposed to a death sentence, our nation has developed myriad weapons to fight HIV diagnoses and HIV-related stigma. Fortunately, these initiatives have often been successful; for example, analysis of the federal government's official HIV information-dissemination website, HIV.gov, revealed that the annual number of HIV infections decreased from 2014 to 2018.[1] In addition, when analyzing figures by age group in that same period, rates of HIV-positive diagnoses decreased for ages 13–24, 35–44, 45–54 and 55+. However, for individuals ages 25–34 the rate remained stable.[2] On first glance, it appears that our tools are reducing HIV diagnoses but that this success is not universal.

Marginalized communities continue to be left in the shadows. Although stories of success are often paraded around, providing an illusion of progress, many demographic groups have yet to see, feel, or experience such progress. This is especially true for Black men who have sex with other men (Black MSM). According to the latest CDC reports, while rates of HIV incidence are declining in other demographic groups, Black MSM are experiencing the opposite: the last decade has ushered in elevated rates of HIV-positive diagnoses. For example, a 2014 White House report released by the Obama administration found a 22 percent increase in HIV incidence among young Black MSM. In a more recent study, Black MSM, especially between the ages of 13–34, were nearly twice as likely as their white counterparts to contract HIV.[3] Of the 38,739 new HIV diagnoses in 2017, 10,070 (37%) of the diagnoses were among Black MSM.[4] Finally, figures released by the 2016 Conference on Retrovirus and Opportunistic Infections (CROI) unveiled a stark projection: if current trends persist, approximately one in two Black MSM will be diagnosed in their lifetime.[5] Such figures highlight a somber but important truth: Black MSM continue to bear the biggest burden in combating HIV.

On July 16, 2012, the U.S. Food and Drug Administration approved Truvada as PrEP to reduce the risk of contracting HIV.[6] Taken once a day, PrEP can decrease the risk of infections by more than 90 percent, and on-demand dosage has also shown promise. Simply put, PrEP is an incredibly robust tool that can be used to decrease HIV.[7] Yet despite its promise and empirically proven results, PrEP has yet to largely reach Black MSM, the community that needs it most. Using a hypothetical scenario/case study approach, this chapter deconstructs the various barriers young Black MSM face in attempting to secure PrEP. Before continuing, it is important to acknowledge that the Black MSM experience is not monolithic; in other words, the scenario presented should not be assumed to be a universal truth for all Black MSM. Instead, I implore you to read it as an illustrative narrative based on research; this story could be (and is) the reality of many young Black MSM across the country. Lastly, as you digest Dante's story, pay close attention to the various assumptions embedded in the biomedical approach to prescribing PrEP.

"I Heard about It Before, but I Don't Know Where to Get It": A Case Study

Dante is a self-identifying gay 21-year-old college junior who attends an historically Black college in the Deep South. Dante comes from a low-income family but was awarded several merit and need-based scholarships. As with many students, his scholarships cover all the "necessities" of college but aren't enough to help Dante with daily living expenses such as toiletries and food. Dante was given a car when he graduated from high school, but it has since broken down and he cannot afford to get it fixed. Therefore, Dante uses the college's and the city's public transit system. Dante works part-time on campus as a resident assistant at his dormitory.

Like many Black gay men growing up in the Deep South, Dante was socialized in a world fueled by racism and homophobia.[8] As a kid, he was teased for having feminine qualities and faced verbal and emotional abuse by family members. Comments like "stop being a sissy," "you're going to hell," and "shit like that is for girls" were commonplace for Dante. Although family members may have treated these as asides or throw-away comments, they were seared into Dante's brain. He internalized them, experiencing crippling internalized homophobia.[9] As Dante grew up, he felt guilt, shame, and fear about his same-sex attraction. He tried to "shut off" his attractions and pretended to be sexually attracted to cis-gender women; such behavior carries multiple negative mental health implications including depression and suicidal ideation.[10] Despite his church's homophobia and homonegativity, like many Black MSM, Dante chose to remain steadfast in his church/faith, seeing religion as an identity anchor.[11] He desperately attempted to "pray the gay away" multiple times, but to no avail.

Dante felt some sense of freedom when he went away to college. For many queer Black youth, college is the first time they feel they can truly be themselves.[12] Dante had his first same-sex encounter as a freshman. At first, Dante was adamant about using condoms every time he had sex with another man. However, Dante falls in love with an older gentleman, who encourages him to "fuck raw." Mixing sexual networks—moving into various networks based on race, age and other differences—is incredibly popular among Black MSM and is a known risk factor for HIV.[13] In an attempt to secure some form of intimacy and comfort, Dante engages in unprotected receptive intercourse ("bottoming") with the older gentlemen. After the encounter, Dante feels guilt and immediately discloses his actions to his friends. He experiences increased stress and anxiety, fearing he has contracted HIV. That night, he and his friends are watching Shonda Rhimes's TV show *How to Get Away with Murder.* A character mentions PrEP in one of the first times the pill is mentioned on a nationwide TV show.[14] Dante intently watches the episode, and a friend tells him, "Oh yeah! I heard about PrEP before." Dante perks up and asks for more information, but no one in the room knows any more about it. His friend adds, "I've heard about it before, but I don't know how to get it." At this point, Dante wants to learn more, but doesn't want to be perceived as promiscuous; many in the community view taking PrEP as irresponsible and reckless, giving individuals an excuse to be slutty.[15]

Dante is at a critical psychological crossroads; he has already overcome his internalized homophobia, but now, he has to go through the mental process of deciding whether he wants to go on PrEP. To some, doing so inherently labels Dante a whore. Dante decides to take total control of his sexual health and embarks on the journey to get on PrEP. Unfortunately, he is about to learn that one's desire to get on PrEP does not always translate to securing the potentially life-changing prescription.

"Just Gonna Make You Have More Sex"

After hearing about PrEP on TV and from one of his friends, Dante desperately wants to learn more about it. However, he is reluctant to use his campus health center because (1) he is afraid of someone finding out about his inquiry, and (2) previous encounters have encouraged Dante to believe the staff may be homophobic. While being treated for flu-like symptoms, Dante overheard a nurse say, "Make sure you give him an HIV test," a microaggression launched at him due to his sexuality.

Dante decides to use the internet to learn more about PrEP. Because of his search history and access to cookies, once he logs onto Facebook, he is bombarded with PrEP-related information. However, all of the information Dante sees is related to the problems with taking PrEP: personal injury advertisements are plastered across his feed.[16] Dante comes across various alleged class action lawsuits documenting horrific side effects, including permanent kidney damage, but he researches further and learns that these stories are a systemic misinformation campaign and that PrEP is relatively safe.[17] Fueled by the desire to take proactive measures, Dante continues his search and learns that he first must locate a provider who is willing to prescribe PrEP. At this point, Dante becomes extremely discouraged because his search yields dismal results. Bernstein writes, "In the South, what he [the subject of Bernstein's article] can't find is PrEP, the once-a-day pill that protects users against HIV infection, or a doctor who knows much about it, or a drugstore that stocks it."[18] Dante thinks he has defied the odds when he finally locates a provider. However, once he gets to the doctor's office, he is disappointed again as the physician subtly shoots down his request. Often, doctors report knowing about PrEP but are reluctant to prescribe it because (1) they "aren't aware of long term effects," and (2) believe it is a pill for promiscuity since it will increase rates of unprotected sex.[19] Research suggests that Dante's problem is at least threefold: he has to find a doctor who is knowledgeable about PrEP, who is willing to prescribe PrEP, and who will not display racism, slut shaming, or homophobia.[20] Although he is discouraged, Dante is now four weeks into his journey to secure PrEP, and like other Black MSM, he finally asks a trusted friend for advice; by word of mouth, Dante learns of a gay-friendly clinic that provides PrEP.[21] Ecstatic, he rushes to his computer to map the route to the clinic. Here, Dante is dealt another devastating blow; the clinic is a forty-five-minute drive away, and ninety minutes via public transit. Lack of transportation is one of the biggest barriers to securing PrEP.[22] With limited income and no car, Dante has to figure out a way to get to the clinic.

Remember that Dante is carrying multiple stressors; his desire to get on PrEP is not his only concern. HIV does not exist in a vacuum but instead augments the stressors one may already face. Dante is a full-time student, carrying the weight of a full course load. Due to limited income and familial circumstances, like many college students, Dante also may face food insecurity or other serious financial hardships.[23] At this point, other individuals might feel burned out and discouraged and never get prescribed PrEP.[24] However, as a highly motivated individual, Dante picks up extra shifts and decides to save up money to pay for a transit pass to the clinic. He accounts for the three-hour transit time but did not account for the long wait time at the clinic. Due to the wait time, Dante misses class on an important day and faces a grade-deduction penalty, bringing him from a B- to a C.

However, despite all the hurdles and negative consequences, Dante finally comes face to face with a doctor who is openly accepting and willing to prescribe PrEP. After going through the traditional intake protocol, the physician assures Dante that he is an ideal candidate for PrEP and can start the regimen once tests have been completed. Dante asks the doctor where and when tests can be done. His stomach drops as he is faced with another common barrier: comprehensive HIV testing is frequently done in a location different from the prescribing doctor's office. Luckily, seeing Dante's despair, the physician agrees to test him on site for his initial consultation. She explains that the prescription will be filled for three months and will only continue if Dante continues to receive comprehensive screenings every three months. Dante happily agrees; he completely understands that traveling to and from the clinic may not be sustainable, but the three-month prescription is a small victory in the larger battle.

Unfortunately, Dante's state of euphoria is short-lived. When he picks up his prescription at the local pharmacy, he is stunned by the price. Someone without insurance drug coverage would pay around $8,000 a year for a year's worth of PrEP.[25] Luckily, because he is under 26, Dante is covered by his mother's insurance, and his prescription comes in at around $90 a month. However, this is still a hefty price tag for a financially independent college student. Dante finds a way to cover the cost of his first month but has no idea how he will cover the additional out-of-pocket costs. Just when Dante is able to gain some sense of peace and comfort, his mom calls him and is furious. In his secret journey to secure PrEP, Dante failed to realize that his mother would receive all the bills, invoices, and all other documentation. She explains that while the visit may have *appeared* free, the family has yet to meet their deductible payment for their health insurance, and therefore, they were billed nearly $550 for the doctor visit alone. The cost of the comprehensive tests is still pending. The call from his mother is like a dagger in his heart; not only has Dante saddled his mother with medical debt but he is also faced with difficult questions related to *what* he was doing at the doctor office and why. Like many young Black MSM, Dante's fortitude and resilience simply aren't enough. Through tears and trembling, he hangs up the phone and decides this will be his first and last month on PrEP. His increased self-efficacy is no match for the systems of oppression at work.

Although dreary, Dante's hypothetical story is the unfortunate reality for many young Black MSM across the country. The purpose of this chapter is not to spread a fatalistic view of PrEP and HIV in the Black MSM community. Instead, it should be viewed as a cautionary tale. The current paradigm for rolling out PrEP is largely predicated on a biomedical approach, relying almost exclusively on increased awareness, self-efficacy, and a heightened locus of control. But this chapter clearly outlines that one may *want* to get and stay on PrEP but still lack the ability to do so. Dante's story most certainly does not have to be the typical tale for a young Black MSM. We must fight systemic inequalities in all forms, but especially related to PrEP. We must fight for men like Dante who struggled and lost, not because he did not know how to box but because he, and many like him, was never invited to the ring.

Notes

1. "U.S. Statistics," HIV.gov, June 30, 2020, https://www.hiv.gov /hiv-basics/overview/data-and-trends/statistics.

2. "U.S Statistics."

3. Centers for Disease Control (CDC), *HIV and African American Gay and Bisexual Men* (Atlanta: Centers for Disease Control and Prevention, June 19, 2020).

4. CDC, *HIV and African American Gay and Bisexual Men.*

5. Liz Highleyman, "Major Disparities Persist in Lifetime Risk of HIV Diagnosis in the US," February 24, 2016. https://www .aidsmap.com/news/feb-2016/major-disparities-persist-lifetime -risk-hiv-diagnosis-us.

6. Matt G. Mutchler, Bryce Mcdavitt, Mansur A. Ghani, Kelsey Nogg, Terrell J. A. Winder, and Juliana K. Soto, "Getting PrEPared for HIV Prevention Navigation: Young Black Gay Men Talk About HIV Prevention in the Biomedical Era," *AIDS Patient Care and STDs* 29, no. 9 (2015): 490–502. doi:10.1089/ apc.2015.0002.

7. Kristen Underhill, Kathleen M. Morrow, Christopher Colleran, Sarah K. Calabrese, Don Operario, Peter Salovey, and Kenneth H. Mayer, "Explaining the Efficacy of Pre-Exposure Prophylaxis (PrEP) for HIV Prevention: A Qualitative Study of Message Framing and Messaging Preferences among US Men Who Have Sex with Men." *AIDS and Behavior* 20, no. 7 (2015): 1514–1526. doi:10.1007/s10461-015-1088-9.

8. Ari Shapiro and Dave Blanchard, "Ending HIV in Mississippi Means Cutting through Racism, Poverty and Homophobia,"

NPR, March 16, 2019. https://www.npr.org/sections/health-shots/2019/03/16/696862618/ending-hiv-in-mississippi-means-cutting-through-racism-poverty-and-homophobia.

9. Katherine Quinn, Julia Dickson-Gomez, Wayne Difranceisco, Jeffrey A. Kelly, Janet S. St. Lawrence, Yuri A. Amirkhanian, and Michelle Broaddus, "Correlates of Internalized Homonegativity among Black Men Who Have Sex with Men," *AIDS Education and Prevention* 27, no. 3 (2015): 212–226. doi:10.1521/aeap.2015.27.3.212.

10. Jeremy J. Gibbs and Jeremy Goldbach, "Religious Conflict, Sexual Identity, and Suicidal Behaviors among LGBT Young Adults," *Archives of Suicide Research* 19, no. 4 (2015): 472–488. https://doi.org/10.1080/13811118.2015.1004476.

11. Quinn et al., "Internalized Homonegativity," 220–221.

12. "'There Is Change Happening': Historically Black Colleges Tackle LGBTQ Rights," *The Guardian*, April 22, 2019.

13. John A. Schneider, Benjamin Cornwell, David Ostrow, Stuart Michaels, Phil Schumm, Edward O. Laumann, and Samuel Friedman, "Network Mixing and Network Influences Most Linked to HIV Infection and Risk Behavior in the HIV Epidemic among Black Men Who Have Sex with Men," *American Journal of Public Health* 103, no. 1 (2013): e28–e36. doi:10.2105/ajph.2012.301003.

14. Allison Piwowarski, "What Is PrEP? Connor's HIV Prevention Pills on 'How to Get Away with Murder' Will Hopefully Keep Him Safe," Bustle, October 9, 2015. https://www.bustle.com/articles/115937-what-is-prep-connors-hiv-prevention-pills-on-how-to-get-away-with-murder-will-hopefully.

15. Alex Dubov, Phillip Galbo, Frederick L. Altice, and Liana Fraenkel, "Stigma and Shame Experiences by MSM Who Take PrEP for HIV Prevention: A Qualitative Study," *American Journal of Men's Health* 12, no. 6 (2018): 1843–1854. doi:10.1177/1557988318797437.

16. Tony Romm, "Facebook Ads Push Misinformation about HIV Prevention Drugs, LGBT Activists Say, 'Harming Public Health,'" *Washington Post*, December 9, 2019.

17. Romm, "Facebook Ads."

18. Lenny Bernstein, "This HIV Pill Saves Lives: So Why Is It so Hard to Get in the Deep South?" *Washington Post*, March 12, 2019.

19. Steven P. Kurtz and Mance E. Buttram, "Misunderstanding of Pre-Exposure Prophylaxis Use among Men Who Have Sex with Men: Public Health and Policy Implications," *LGBT Health* 3, no. 6 (2016): 461–464. doi:10.1089/lgbt.2015.0069.

20. Andrew E. Petroll, Jennifer L. Walsh, Jill L. Owczarzak, Timothy L. Mcauliffe, Laura M. Bogart, and Jeffrey A. Kelly, "PrEP Awareness, Familiarity, Comfort, and Prescribing Experience among US Primary Care Providers and HIV Specialists," *AIDS and Behavior* 21, no. 5 (2016): 1256–1267. doi:10.1007/s10461-016-1625-1.

21. Mutchler et al., "Getting PrEPared for HIV Prevention Navigation."

22. Liesl A. Nydegger and Kasey R. Claborn, "Exploring Patterns of Substance Use among Highly Vulnerable Black Women at Risk for HIV through a Syndemics Framework: A Qualitative Study," *PLOS ONE* 15, no. 7 (2020). doi:10.1371/journal.pone.0236247.

23. Devon C. Payne-Sturges, Allison Tjaden, Kimberly M. Caldeira, Kathryn B. Vincent, and Amelia M. Arria, "Student Hunger on Campus: Food Insecurity among College Students and Implications for Academic Institutions," *American Journal of Health Promotion* 32, no. 2 (2017): 349–354. doi:10.1177/0890117117719620.

24. Mutchler et al., "Getting PrEPared for HIV Prevention Navigation."

25. Emma Sophia Kay and Rogério M. Pinto, "Is Insurance a Barrier to HIV Preexposure Prophylaxis? Clarifying the Issue," *American Journal of Public Health* 110, no. 1 (2020): 61–64. doi:10.2105/ajph.2019.305389.

8

PrEP in the Porn World

PAM DORE, AKA MR. PAM

The porn industry argued about HIV for many years. The straight porn industry never officially adopted condoms, but they tested their performers regularly. If you were HIV-positive or had an STI you couldn't work. The state of California tried to require condoms throughout the industry, but the whole industry just got up and moved to Las Vegas. The gay side mostly used condoms until the late 1990s. But since 2012 PrEP has revolutionized the gay porn industry. Truvada and Descovy have not only transformed the adult industry but also gay sex in general.

I first heard of PrEP around 2009 when one of my models started on a drug trial. He was the ultimate 21-year-old power-bottom, not only getting pounded on screen often but also many of his nights out turned into weekend cruising for dick in the bathhouses and underground sex clubs of New York City. He would go on binges, his butthole insatiable—and if HE was still negative, then WOW! This shit really works!

Fast-forward to 2012: after gay men starting using PrEP, they began having all the sex they wanted: it was like birth control for gay men. A pill once a day and no HIV! So, after years of men swearing by this medication and with testing also becoming a lot more popular and accessible, the floodgates were open and bareback–the nonviral-load-weekend version—took off. Testing procedures in the gay industry (following the straight industry) were becoming more common among gay porn companies; before that it was more of "slap a condom on and don't ask, don't tell" about your HIV status because, yes, using condoms for the prevention of HIV transmission does work and had worked for years— it didn't feel good, it killed boners, but at least it worked. So after PrEP came along, the gay porn industry was charging up to abandon their "wrap it up" policy and entering the world of testing: giving PrEP for negative models and testing for "undetectable" status for positive models.

Currently, HIV and STI testing takes place at a network of Talent Testing facilities scattered around the United States. The green "CLEAR" alert has become the standard of model safety and STD prevention. It's not cheap: a test will run between $180 to $225 and is good for two weeks to work. And it's not foolproof—a lot of sexual activity can happen for some men in a two-week window, letting the dick-colds or clap (gonorrhea) sneak through. But models are becoming more careful about the kind of sex they have offset, knowing that sex with "civilians" can cost them thousands of dollars if they test positive. Luckily the stigma of having HIV or catching a "dick-cold," which comes with being a porn model or sex worker, has greatly subsided. Dick-colds just suck for everyone, and we will do anything to avoid them.

HIV in gay porn is easily manageable with modern testing and medication. The testing facilities can now test a model's T-cell count and determine his or her "undetectable" status. Models who are on PrEP or who are educated about status levels are happy to film with a sero-discordant scene partner. And even better—the "don't ask, don't tell" unwritten/unofficial policy of gay porn of the past has had the gag ripped off, and open discussion and education around HIV transmission are now encouraged.

Of course, the gay porn industry strives to create hot scenes for fans to watch and enjoy—but keeping the performers healthy and safe is the most important goal. Creating porn with guidelines and safety protocols makes a better product: models feel safer on set to explore their sexuality, try new things, demonstrate the old, and have a blast. Directors and camera crews feel better knowing that everyone is tested and they don't have to be vigilant, watching a condom to determine whether it's getting too stretchy or worn down and needs to be changed, or gawd-forbid it breaks. And fans get the benefit of a hot bareback sex scene!

However, there are some negative things about PrEP. It's really hard on your body, and it's a lot to handle for performers who only have sex on camera with tested performers. A lot of guys are not on PrEP now because of its negative effects on the liver; those who are also pushing the limits with body-enhancing supplements (steroids . . . shhhh) don't take it. So, unless they're super gay and at the bathhouse or blowing up Grindr, they're choosing not to be on PrEP. My partner Ricky, who is a performer in gay adult films, and I are not on PrEP. I tried it but it made me very sick. I also didn't trust the testing. I know it's still risky and STDs still occasionally sneak in, but we still choose not to be on PrEP. Recently, my boyfriend filmed a scene with one of our really great friends, who has been open about being HIV-positive. It was Ricky's first bareback scene with a positive performer. We did a long interview with the performer before we shot the scene and talked about the stigma and testing. Ricky then did the scene. It was hot!

9

Auto-Pharmakon

Prescribing Utopia

ADDISON VAWTERS

1. In 1988, ACT UP activists laid siege to the Food and Drug Administration. In 1996 they dumped the ashes of their dead lovers on the White House lawn. Storming the National Institutes of Health in 1990 was a pivotal moment; shortly thereafter, collaboration between activists, government, and pharmaceutical companies was established. By the late 1990s the activists had taken seats at the boardroom table where they participated in crafting legislation and corporate policy in cooperation with pharmaceutical companies. Even now discourse on HIV research is posed in terms of collaboration with corporate and government scientists, as though they're apolitical technicians with no stake in the issue, when their labor is actually at the heart of it. Their efforts focus on strategic, incremental, and immediate demands on the state, rather than on a transformation of the production of health itself.

2. Although in retrospect it is easy to understand ACT UP's political trajectory considering the group's occupational

and class composition, it is disappointing to acknowledge
that a group congealing around the mantra "Drugs into
Bodies," propelled by hot, righteous love and indignation,
didn't pursue or evolve a more radical program.

3. Militant AIDS activism dissolved at the point where the
liberal and technocratic interplay between corporate and
government management and activist demands had
obtained access to treatment for a predictably privileged
sliver of the population. ACT UP's efforts in citizens'
science are instructive, however, for ongoing and future
political imagining and action.

4. Almost by design, patents kill—by exclusion of less
profitable lifesaving remedies. A pharmaceutical patent is
a necropolitical legal form operating at the nexus of the
state and the corporation. The state's power over life and
death is extended to the corporation through a regulatory
agreement protecting the corporation's right to profit,
based on a philosophically bereft intellectual property
regime. The right to prevent others from producing and
distributing lifesaving products is granted to the inventor,
although often after massive public investment in the
research leading to the discovery. Although this arrange-
ment is heinous enough, the process by which corporations select which drugs to produce also operates on an
exclusionary principle, abandoning populations that die
and those whose ailments aren't profitable. Omitted from
this system entirely is experimental drug discovery for
purposes of the expansion of mental, physical, and sexual
pleasure.

5. Chemicals that help us attain some of these ends
(synthetic hormones and pre-exposure prophylaxes, to
name a few) were discovered in the course of public
research. But queer life is indebted every day to an industry
that only makes pharmaceuticals available by virtue of

their profitability. The fabulous sums earned by the pharmaceutical companies result in a tax on the exploration of gender, on pleasure, on promiscuity, and basically on our subjective potential. Who we are is at stake. The pharmaceutical subject is the result of this miserable economic relation between the industry and the state.

6. If we prefigure a future at least as life-giving as what we have now, then synthetic hormones and PrEP are essential components of sexual, gender, and political liberation. Moreover, liberation requires access to the means of drug discovery, the autonomous selection of which drugs are produced, and which dimensions of gender, sexual, and mental subjectivity are to be explored. This speculative project of autonomous production is a process of resistance, named by Paul Preciado as "techno somatic communism."

7. Meth producers, people who use recreational drugs, steroid users, and users of sex hormones are even now working collectivity in autonomous networks of production and distribution, creating and exchanging chemicals at local and international scales.

8. Postrevolutionary utopian visions frequently rely on pastoral, antediluvian fantasies where trans people, the promiscuous, and the disabled couldn't possibly exist, nor those living with high blood pressure, depression, HIV, or Hep-C. Prevailing theories of libertarian socialist economics, popularly practiced in actually existing autonomous territories, also seem unequipped so far to support the infirm or the cyborg.

9. Upending the current method of pharmaceutical production—and its hold on the production of subjectivity—would require profound transformation, given that pharma industrialists would never relinquish such a productive profit machine easily. Currently, the

pharmaceutical industry prioritizes drugs for treating more profitable chronic diseases over less profitable preventive drugs, leaving many potentially treatable diseases and many possible sexual, psychological, and somatic experiences off the table.

10. The existing open-source pharma movement is for the moment merely a technocratic coalition focused primarily on developing new technological platforms for drug discovery. It must prepare to go far, far beyond to imagine new modes of open- source production and distribution.

11. In the event that pharmaceutical autonomy occurs as part of a broader revolutionary or transformational break, then pharmaceuticals will need to be produced using decentralized and distributed methods.

12. The Autonomous Administration of North and East Syria (NES), also known as Rojava, a de facto autonomous region in northeastern Syria with direct democratic ambitions based on an anarchistic, feminist, and libertarian socialist ideology, produces healthy citizens through the practice of broad public education and participation in health care systems. However, as an unrecognized entity at odds with various regional governments, advanced health care and treatment are unavailable.

Los Municipios Autónomos Rebeldes Zapatistas, de facto autonomous territories founded and controlled by the neo-Zapatista support bases in the Mexican state of Chiapas, are organized around democratic, cooperative, and collective ownership of land and commerce. These zones offer high-quality universal health care with an emphasis on sexual health, funded through economic participation in international markets.

Both political projects, mired in asphyxiating political conflicts with bloodthirsty neighboring states and multinationals, are unable to achieve the level of specialized health care required to sustain the pharmaceutically queer subject. If these innovative projects are to succeed in what would need to be decentralized and democratized pharmaceutical production, a primary activity would need to be the creation of a common pharmaceutical infrastructure, including machinery, constituent chemicals and reactants, and testing protocols.

13. Modern pharmaceutical firms have developed sophisticated powers of production, organizational management, and quality control operating at impressive scales and using extremely specialized knowledge and equipment. Autonomous or commons-based pharma will require the same infrastructure. To illustrate, BioCubaFarma, Cuba's common biotechnology and pharmaceutical firm, has 21,000 employees, covering a continuum of high-technology process specialists. Communities will be called on to deliberate on what scale of production is necessary and then arrange to procure rare minerals, urinary estrogen, and the water rights required for the production processes. Geographic access to resources is unevenly distributed across the globe. To achieve scientific and technological goals, autonomous zones will have to be innovative and determine interzonal trade relations.

14. Although there is nothing inherently revolutionary about being gay now, it will take a revolution to wrest the means of both industrial production and the production of subjectivity from the pharma industry and the enabling state. Soon, surely, under the ongoing pharmacological regime of neglect and death, queer political horizons will be reinvigorated with a renewed sense of militant imagination.

Perspective
Trauma and Healing

Out gay male and lesbian communities had existed for barely more than decade when HIV was discovered. Although gay and bisexual men were initially the most directly affected, in the long run, the epidemic imposed large-scale cumulative harm on the entirety of LGBTQ communities. Yet, the effect of the historical trauma of AIDS has been double-edged. On the one hand, HIV and the problematics of transmission and prevention have brought awareness of gay male sexuality and especially anal intercourse into public view at a level completely unimaginable before HIV. On the other hand, the preeminence of the political battles in late 1990s and 2000s over marriage equality led LGBTQ activists to downplay the rich perversities of queer desire. It has encouraged a kind of domestication of homosexual eroticism and its incorporation into marital scripts.

What are the emotional and personal issues at stake in dealing with changing sexual practices during the AIDS crisis and afterward? How have gay men dealt with challenges to the emotional and psychological significance of their sexual lives in the context of racial, gender, and class inequalities?

During the darkest days of the crisis, gay men not only had to assess the significance of anal intercourse in general but also had to decide whether to abandon the widely held "egalitarian" preference during the 1970s for sexual "versatility"—of moving back and forth from being the one penetrating to the one being penetrated. As awareness of the mode of transmission grew, for example, a more rigid distinction emerged in gay pornographic films between performers playing "top" and "bottom." Understanding the place of anal intercourse in gay men's sex lives is important not only because, as epidemiologists discovered, it is one of the most efficient means of transmitting HIV. Anal sex is considered by many gay men to be one of the most valued aspects of their sexuality—for both the pleasure it yields and the complicated meanings it may have regarding gender roles, subjectivity, and relationality.

During the AIDS crisis, survival—not merely physical but also cultural and sexual—was at stake. Yet the trauma of an epidemic did not negate our need to be touched, to connect, to feel desire. In today's new era of gay sexuality, we are figuring out where things fit, why we want the things we do, and what's possible.

Sex can be healing. Another's touch reveals our bodies to us, the pressure in unfamiliar places, the titillation of discovery, the sensation of a tongue or a hand or a foot. The geography of the neck, the ear, the arm. The taste of skin, tongue, ass, balls, armpits. The smells. Some find they want more, that pushing their bodies in a direction can help silence the constant stream of anxieties, worries, and concerns. The limits of rationality and selfhood are revealed in the moment. Our desires can reveal what we won't or can't face or articulate: we want more.

10

S(t)imulation

LORE/TTA LEMASTER

The town, a simulation in the Baudrillardian sense, is hyperreal—attempting to capture a romanticized moment that loosely parallels the late nineteenth-century Klondike Gold Rush that drew more than 100,000 white terrorist settlers into Tlingit land, of whom roughly 30,000 completed the dangerous trek. Today, the town is vibrant, colorful, a tourist trap. It is at the racist edge of so-called civilization. And I am that: a tourist, reluctantly joining bio-fam in their quest for an "authentic" Alaskan vacation, our first and only "family vacation," to be certain. It's me and two cishet couples: a fat hairy trans femme and four normative cishets who routinely project fear onto my exceptional gender, sexuality, and body. I cannot help but wonder: If we had the funds to secure a trip of this sort when I was younger, would I have accepted the illusion with greater ease, consuming the carefully curated narrative that dulls colonial terror's edge or that lures me in with the violent curiosity of the settler's gaze and an open wallet? In any event, I am here now, a femme faggot with critical tools that render the scene underwhelming, frustrating. And my wallet is empty. I am here because *they* are paying in an attempt to make me feel "included"—although inclusion on their terms feels like shit.

They hurl unprovoked, public insults under the auspices of care:

> You're a fucking man!
>> "Mister" is a compliment!
>>> Why can't you just be gay?!
>>>> "They" isn't a pronoun!
>>>> What am I supposed to do about your gender?!
>>>> You'd make an ugly woman!

The thing is this: I abandoned "family" years ago, when I learned cishet love was conditional, manipulative, violent as fuck. I don't remember when I last genuinely invested in bio-fam. To reiterate: I am here because *they* are paying in an attempt to make me feel "included." And the turmoil is but the bio-fam tax I must pay in the form of affective disconnection, thousands of miles from my partners and t4t sweeties, and covered in drab clothing coded for so-called men—it's my hell simulated.

I step down a side street, as the sexy femme budtender directed, where seasonal tourist industry workers reside and who have, over time, become "the locals" even if seasonal, further displacing indigeneity. The sexy femme budtender cautions, "It's legal, but you can't smoke in public. So, take side streets and act like you live here."

"And where do you live?" I inquire, grabbing the pre-packed joint, holding her gaze.

Her left brow arches—she hadn't read the depths of my queerness—as she stands up straight, taller than me. "Just around the corner. I get off in fifteen." She shifts the dynamic and takes control of my gaze, scanning my bearded femme body. "How about you? Wanna get off in fifteen, too?"

Her voice is hot gravel that melts my heart to life. And I feel. I clarify, "Just so you know, I'm trans."

She retorts without pause, "Yeah, me, too. I don't fuck with cissies, boo." My edge softens to meet her intensity. She adds, "And I want my femme cock deep inside of you." She bites her rouged lip as I pivot and walk toward the door, the old wooden floor creaking underfoot.

I reach for the handle and pull the door open, looking back over my shoulder at the sexy femme budtender, "See you in fifteen." A faint waft of cannabis escapes the bar behind me along with an excited giggle.

The white cishet family, a simulation in the Baudrillardian sense, is hyperreal—attempting to capture while violently asserting a romanticized relational modality that traffics in racist cisheteronormative discourses, logics, aesthetics, and sensibilities. The "family" is a hegemonic trap constituted through exclusion at the edge of so-called civilization.

In short, it is extraordinarily boring and exceptionally stultifying.

The door closes behind me as I exhale, letting my cool-queer façade fade and, along with it, my stature, allowing my big, soft, hairy belly to expand and fall back to its usual posture over my belt. I smile, head to the left, step down a side street as the sexy femme budtender directed, and light up my joint. I pause and inhale, the smoke reaching down deep.

My lungs expand and
I feel my body.
    numb.
        dissociation fades.

And with it
    hyperreal
        familial and
        bodily
        intelligibility and
        worth.
Whhhhhhewwwwwwwwwwwwwwwwwwwwwwwww-
    www
I exhale *and* release
    familial simulation
and crave corporeal stimulation.
To be
felt feeling.

"Of course, I've seen *The Matrix*. What kind of trans femme do you take me for!" I exclaim, flirting. We are lying on either side of an old worn-out couch, something she "inherited" from the prior tenant who inherited it from the prior tenant and so on. It's ugly but comfortable against my bare skin.

She looks up at me and responds coyly, "Look. I don't know. We did *just* meet." Her strong hands caress my feet while she relentlessly teases the head of my small clit with her toes; again. Her now flaccid femme cock lies against the inside of her thigh, atop a puddle of lube and cum and me.

"Um, it's been *at least* an hour," I retort laughing; she follows just behind me.

"Clearly long enough to explore your depths. A few times."

Our laughter slows, and I respond, "Fuck. Thank you, again. It's nice to simply feel and be felt."

"Yeah, bio-fam can be the worst. Plus, I really wanted to feel your fat hairy femme body while I can."

I giggle, like I do. "Why did you ask me about *The Matrix*?"

"Oh, right! You know that whole scene with Morpheus where he says something like 'take the blue pill and believe whatever you want but take the red pill and you stay in Wonderland.'"

"Yeah, I call it the Wachowskian dichotomy." She stares disappointingly at me. "Yeah, it's not my best work."

"Clearly." We both laugh. She continues, "Well, look, if *The Matrix* is a trans allegory, and the red pill signifies gender liberation and what not, then what does this blue pill signify?" She holds up a small blue rectangle GSI 225 pill: Descovy.

"Well, let's not get too literal."

"I mean, Premarin was commonly used for HRT in the 1990s. It was red."

"Huh." I blink contemplatively, having never explored the allegory's depth but just sticking to the surface.

"One pill facilitates agentic gender expression while the other pill facilitates agentic sexual expression."

"I think your agentic sexual expression is slipping out of my agentic gender expression right now." We both return to laughing.

"The point is this," her toes still tickling the head of my small clit, "does the blue pill also enable complacency with sexual oppression against our queer and trans siblings who are living with HIV, detectable *and* not?"

I add, "Does it separate us from ourselves?"

"Not based on the alleged claim that my sexual agency is oozing out of you. Perhaps it's time for one more go before you have to head back to your silly voyage at sea."

"Yes, please. It's the only thing that feels real."

I trek back across the small town and to the large ship that will take us off to our next simulated destination. The town and the cishet family I am returning to are simulations in the Baudrillardian sense—hyperreal constructs attempting to capture, while violently asserting, relational modalities that work in the service of perpetuating advanced capitalism's façade of normality secured through exclusion.

I manage to make it back to my cabin unseen. I order room service to be delivered in thirty minutes, giving me time to prepare for the quick descent into sleep just after food. I undress from the day, slipping into a long silk lavender robe. I strategically wash my face, avoiding my beard—I want to smell the sexy femme budtender's body on my beard tomorrow amidst the ebb and flow of bio-familial terror. I reach into my toiletry bag to retrieve my medications: an SSRI, Omeprazole, and Descovy.

> Queer worlds are devised of small devices.
>> Little pills,
>>> blue and red.
>> Enabling
>>> a fleeting felt sense of feeling, being, and becoming
>>>> alive. Together.

11

Playing in the Shadows

Cycles of Trauma

ARIEL SABILLON

I come to the following ideas as an immigrant, a Honduran, and a queer. Because of these identities, much of my life has been framed by fleeing violence. My journey through sex has been in the context of the 2000s, and I tested positive for HIV in high school. When I was in college, someone filed a case against me at the university because I did not disclose my HIV status before having oral sex with him in the dorms. I might have been expelled, and the entire process left me feeling unsupported, targeted, and marginalized at my college. After graduating, I traveled and met people and engaged in different healing practices to make sense of these experiences.

These are some thoughts about healing and sex within the contexts of HIV, culture, immigration, masculinity, and femininity. What follows is a transcription of a conversation I had with Andrew Spieldenner.

HIV is a symptom of an entire network of illnesses. If we alleviate HIV as a symptom, whether through antiretrovirals

(ARVs) or a cure, it does not necessarily mean we have treated the root cause of the illness. It is an illness of sexuality, and we don't have a society that promotes healthy sexuality.

Humans need to build trusting communities with strong foundations based on shared values. We've become separated and isolated from each other. For HIV to be fully healed, and not have another illness take its place, we must be in communion with one another. If I were to get into a car crash, and the doctor merely treated my broken arm without addressing head damage, cuts, and scratches, that would be considered negligent. The same applies to our response to HIV. HIV is inextricably linked to other diseases and challenges us at both a community and a global level.

HIV has been part of the way that I interact in my relationships with romantic and sexual partners and the way that I relate to myself. In my high school and early college years, I was not very conscious of the way that I had sex. I was having sex in a very dangerous way. It was spiritually dangerous and reckless; it was unconscious. It made for a crazy environment and stirred up a lot of negative feelings within myself and with my sexual partners.

Now I ask myself, What do I want sexually? I heard someone on a podcast ask if pornography or sex work can be spiritual. The answer is a definitive "yes!" Spiritual sex work depends on the consciousness and intention behind it. To pursue this spiritual dimension of sex, I needed to access a "feminine" power because I feel more of a feminine, rather than masculine, energy. However, I misunderstood what it meant to be feminine when I used sexual seduction as a tool of manipulation. It wasn't healthy. A couple of weeks ago, I decided I wanted sex again, and I actually started being sexual and intimate with a guy in a vulnerable way. We were engaging with each other on multidimensional levels. It felt amazing. I discovered that sex can be an amazing tool for connection—for connecting with myself and for connecting with my partners.

Ever since we were born, we were made for sex and sensuality. Recognizing that as a daily part of my life has been liberatory. When a guy doesn't text me back in two days, I think, "I thought we were going to have sex with each other and be in a relationship." But I know this fantasy wasn't even about that guy: my desire was for a connection with people, a physical connection with people.

I'm a sexual being who enjoys having sex. I feel like I lost that part of me when I was accused of hiding my HIV-positive status from my sex partner. I thought, "I am going to jail." My trial and the way the university handled it really threw me off. I felt like I couldn't healthily engage with sex. I wanted to be in a relationship—to be with just the one partner—because then I don't have to worry about disclosing my status and facing social ostracization. Sometimes, it is unclear to me if I am seeking a spiritual connection or a purely physical connection with another person. I'm open to a relationship, but I'm also open to three-day relationships.

Sex is a primal energy; it's what animates your life force. Even if you only know your sex partner for that one night or for that one week or for the rest of your life, it doesn't matter! It is still a divine union, and I'm ready to step into that power.

A couple of years ago, my ex posted a video of us having sex on social media. I look so cute in it. I wasn't mad because I looked back at it, and damn! I was getting railed! It reminded me of a part of myself that I missed after my trial—the little feisty part. Am I holding some resentment about the video? I think I would be embarrassed if he posted it now, but at that time in my life, mostly gay men followed me. So, I wasn't worried about the exposure.

Now I think that there was a sinister aspect to posting our sex video. He had done that before—to a seventeen-year-old—and was charged with having child pornography. I looked him up after our relationship ended and found his mugshot and an article about him. The article quotes him insisting he did nothing wrong because this person liked being videotaped. When I knew him, this man probably had the sexual maturity of a 14-year-old when it came to sex. He was not mature enough to take responsibility. The law got involved and criminalized him.

But there was a loop there that kept repeating. He came to me because I play the little boy sometimes; that's what he likes. I felt shame about how I got involved with him on these terms. We want to keep running away from the unseemly and unsettling aspects of sexual desire. The media and the law would write off this man as a pedophile, preventing us from looking deeper into his suffering and the reasons why he may inflict suffering on others through illegal sexual play. If we run away from it, if we don't face it, then it's going to keep happening. We have to come from a place of nonjudgment and open up that book. When we run away from it, the more those loops keep coming up. I'm playing that loop out of shame, fear, and guilt about my desires, but I understand these feelings don't originate inside me. They came from somebody else. I've bought into a story that is not mine. These destructive patterns and feelings are not mine but have been passed down from previous relationships and inflect the way I relate to others in the present. I can let them go, and I don't have to do more about it because they're not mine. Now, I can create a different narrative.

I'm ready now to enjoy a different kind of relationship with a man or woman. I want a relationship where both of us are engaged in a very conscious way and approach each other from a shared point of vulnerability. Sexuality isn't easy, but it's okay to like what you like. We all like a favorite body shape or part. It is not great when shame and guilt intersect in sexuality. Shaming should have no place in sexuality. I can exercise agency with my sexuality, rather than repeating destructive loops.

My experiences as a refugee child inform my feelings of shame. When your family is running from something, you know that things are worse somewhere else. Being part of a community that has gone through massive trauma—death, brutality, murder, gangs, and war—has an impact on your sexual practices and relationships. You start associating with the pain. I understand what goes on in this life, what goes on in this world, and I am so thankful for what we do have because it could be so much worse—it is a lot worse for a lot of different people, as it was for my family and ancestors.

I was able to face up to these horrors because I've made peace, even if this peace is tenuous at best. I'm aware that terrible things happen all the time. When I visited a mass grave in Honduras, I looked at it and thought, "We are not addressing this loss as a community." People don't want to address it because it's painful. I understand where that comes from, but I want to address it.

I have the strength to do so. My spirituality and the way that I look at life are shaped by hunters. Being in those environments gave me strength. I can face great adversity because I have witnessed extreme violence and loss. There were people in my neighborhood who were beheaded. I'm not going to pretend it didn't happen. But at the same time, I am not going to get stuck on the reaction to the horror. I try to observe and then decide whether there is action to be taken because sometimes there isn't anything a single person can do to confront evil.

I believe humans are multidimensional beings, and we're becoming aware of that more and more thanks to the theoretical developments in quantum physics. I feel like this is an overlooked part of human knowledge throughout time, but repressive forces like Christian programming and the inhibitive aspects of shame make us afraid of our power. Sometimes I wonder why I am capable of confronting the darkest aspects of human existence. Regardless, I have accepted taking on this darkness so that I can transmute it and start navigating other ways to live.

In other words, I found happiness when I was able to look at the darkness.

12

When We Touch

A Reading on Queer Intimacies

JUSTICE JAMAL JONES AND
ANDREW SPIELDENNER

Page of Wands: Discovery, Free Spirit

We are two queer men of color from different generations. One of us is more comfortable meeting others in bars; the other came out in the age of apps. We meet to talk in the midst of three interlocking moments: the Trump presidency, the COVID-19 pandemic, and the rise of the Movement for Black Lives. Each of these has affected how we interact and engage with our public and private worlds.

JUSTICE: 2016 was a huge year for change for me. In the traditional tarot card deck, it would be best characterized by the "wheel of fortune," a card that symbolizes cycles and patterns, and change that is out of the hands of the beholder. 2016, with the election of Trump, showed me that for much of my life I had been living in irregularity within the Obama era, where my president looked like me, marriage equality was normal, and Beyoncé was the queen of the world. Trump's election introduced me and many other young people to a cycle that we had thought was old-fashioned, when in fact the Trump presidency was in our cards all along.

The "wheel of fortune" card came to me the first time on a chilly fall freshman year hookup with a much older NYU faculty member. Like many "intellectual" white, queer folk I would soon come across, he claimed to possess mystical powers. His were through the art of tarot. Wide-eyed, fresh, and a bit drunk, I believed him. From what I can remember he pulled me a three-card reading consisting of the "Page of Wands," "Five of Wands," and, of course, the "Wheel of Fortune." I question the accuracy of this post-sex, drunk reading, but do know that the reading was right about fate. Being the young page, fresh to New York, it would be my fate to be caught in a cycle of dating men too old for me who thought they were magical.

ANDREW: 2016 was a year of change for me too. One seven-year relationship ended. Badly. Involving blood and fists and police and threats. "No one will ever love you: you're ugly, you're old, you're fat," my ex tells me. From there, I met a man—much younger—at an academic event. I was smitten that someone so beautiful would find me attractive. We went on a few dates. We laughed. A lot. We made out and slept in the same bed, doing bumps of coke and drinking. He introduced me to Molly. This seemed good.

After a few months, it became obvious the sex wasn't happening. At least not the way either of us wanted. We did not talk about it. Instead, we did more Molly, or coke, or liquor. We got into an easy routine. Every Friday, after he went to the bathhouse, he would come over to my place and I would cook. After, we would head out—sometimes

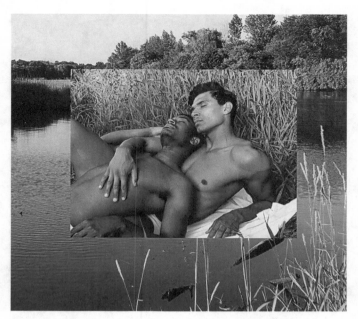

Creative Director: Justice Jamal Jones; Photography: Byron Gamble

to a bar, sometimes to the Cock. We would wake up the next day, go to have breakfast, and called it love. The easy exchanges, the shared humor, the bright smiles, and the mutual admiration made it seem like it could be. I could not connect with him, though, because the bruises of the last relationship were still fresh.

How did we find each other in these spaces? Since 2016, we have gone through moves, made art, and worked on finding a voice and a community, all while surviving a government that is increasingly hostile to Black and brown people, immigrants, queer and trans people, and cis women. We found each other through publications, social media, and Justice's intention to open doors and connect. We write this in the context of the global pandemic of COVID-19 and the end

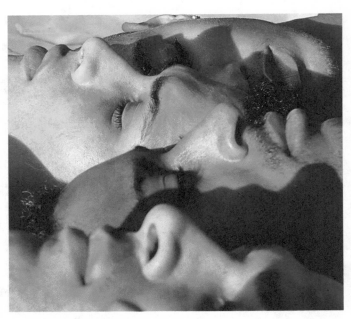

Creative Director: Justice Jamal Jones; Photography: Byron Gamble

of Trump's presidency. We have been forced into isolation: it has been months since we have felt free to touch.

Five of Wands: Conflict, Tension, Opposition

The anxiety is new for some people: those who have never had to be worried about disease when meeting others. The fear of the unknown, the specter of risk rises up and leads them to panic—grabbing shelves of toilet paper, scurrying away from strangers, heart beating faster as someone looms closer. We are familiar with this feeling: every time we approach a man in a bar, on the street, online, we have learned there is risk. *Will he hurt me? Will he like me? Do I tell him about me? Does he have HIV or any STIs? What does he*

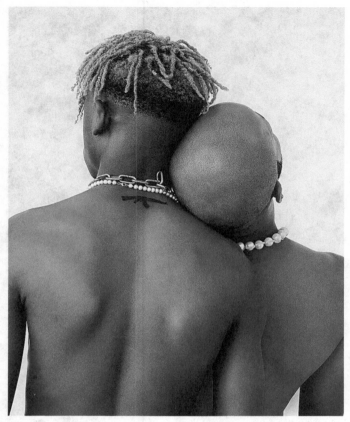

Creative Director: Justice Jamal Jones; Photography: Heather Hooton

want out of this exchange? What do I? These are questions that undergird our Black and brown queer lives.

Online apps have become ubiquitous in our lives. The profiles carry a plethora of data points: what you look like, where you live, what your medical conditions are, what you're into, and sometimes what you're not. There is no privacy: the other users glean as much information as they want (even if

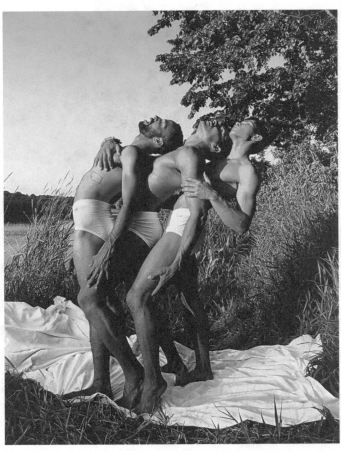

Creative Director: Justice Jamal Jones; Photography: Byron Gamble

some of that is a projection) before ever finding out a name or hearing a voice.

In gay bars, the competition is fierce. Every gay man seems to believe he's famous. The smells of alcohol, musk, cologne, and the smoke machine evoke a posture, preparing to compete for attention, for that look or that man who

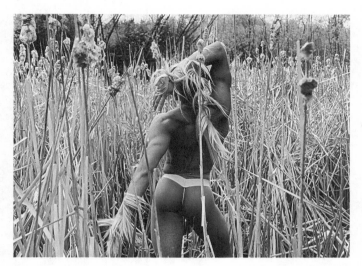
Creative Director: Justice Jamal Jones; Photography: Byron Gamble

indicates you are doing it right. What are we competing for? What do we want? The one-night stand is the one-night stand is the one-night stand. Rinse, repeat. What more is there?

JUSTICE: Like the tarot card of the "Five of Wands," my new role as "sexy black page," fresh to NYC, put me in a certain gay weight class that perpetuated extreme competition. Blinded by insecurity, I took part in such frivolous acts of dominance as thirst trapping on social media or sneaking underage into clubs to compete for attention from men too old for me, which usually led to inappropriate, aggressive sex and heartache.

I have not always been the victim. I have been the villain on occasion, when stealing boyfriends or hate fucking an ex, all acts that made me feel big or grown. But I had to show off my wand. I had to show all the boys what it could do, and I wanted to see their wands; there were so many to try. Or at least that's what I was told. . . .

I'm exhausted. I need more than casual, drunk, messy sex. I want someone who cares. And maybe the person I am waiting for is me? Am I a prude? I don't want to be a part of the Five of Wands. What does the Five of Wands mean? It's intimate but not tender. Sometimes violence can pretend to be a sort of intimacy. At least I am being touched? I'm being noticed? Was it really an embrace or was it a suffocation?

ANDREW: I was lucky to have a couple of older gay men in my life who gave me advice and did not try to sleep with me. They listened, they scolded, they told me about their lives. They let me be a mess; they were proud of what I accomplished and recognized what I had survived. When I meet younger men now, I have to remember the value of being in that role. That maybe they do not want to have sex with me; it's just the first thing they're taught to do to get attention, to get invited in. And to be honest, the attention from these brilliant young people is alluring.

Gay culture is a place of belonging with all its rude and catty ways. The search for intimacy and connection has become more complicated in the pandemic. Finding others to share space with presents challenges when travel and touch are considered risky and a threat to public health. We found each other through acts of writing: reading published work, typing on social media. The networks that encourage our meetings are comprised of multiple competing platforms: the neoliberal university we both currently inhabit, the usage of new media in our everyday ways of being, and the gay community that scripts our interactions as always potential-sex.

Wheel of Fortune: Lifecycles, a Turning Point

We have adjusted the ways that we are intimate. Communities do change: HIV has had—and continues to have—an extraordinary impact on LGBTQ communities globally. Through the years, the community has gone from pushing condoms to encouraging a range of prevention options, from organizing support and political groups to building clinics. There's so much more to health: Black and brown people need to grow and thrive. What happens when we dream? It is so easy to see us as questionable and limited: unable. We accept that our lives have meaning, that we exist. We search for more. We build a future for us to be together.

JUSTICE: At my ripe age of twenty-one years old, I'm done with fucking. Who's to say that I won't have a hookup here and there, but I'm sure not getting fucked, fucked over, or fucked up about men who cannot be intimate.

In fact, who says that it has to be men. On my journey, I have found that the conception of my sexuality preceded my found understanding of gender, which limited my identity. I was given the opportunity to explore my sexuality, spilling my energy and giving my body onto others, but more intimate personal experiences, such as gender, were forgotten. Like the Yoruba God Obatala, I am both male and female, for I am neither. I crave sex and intimacy: I am love.

In much of my journey into adulthood I have been given readings. Readings by men trying to seduce me, or simply being told who I am by those who seek to control me. But I have decided to make my own magic or look to the magic of my ancestors. For what I have found is that I am the holder of my destiny. I am my own wheel of fortune.

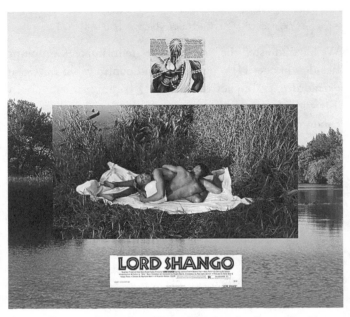

Creative Director: Justice Jamal Jones; Photography: Byron Gamble

The photo essay that accompanies this piece demonstrates some of that world-building. Based on the relationship between Orishas Shango and Obatala of the Yoruba and Santeria spiritualities, "Shango x Obatala" is a digital shrine to the dangerously beautiful intimacy between Black and brown men. Obatala, the child of God, creator of the lands and waters, and father of Shango, is genderless. "His" asexuality makes him the God of all of the human race, regardless of identity. Obatala is associated with the colors white, silver, and ivory.

Shango, their son, is God of war, fire, and lightning. He possesses superhuman strength and stamina, and he often represents the sexuality and vitality of men. His powers are said to be only surpassed by those of Obatala. According to Yoruba tradition, Shango was often misunderstood for his fire, power, and light: these were often mistaken as violence. It took Obatala to step in and give Shango balance and to cool his fire. Obatala can provide asexual love, a position that can give perspective for growth. Their relationship is cyclical, and we can learn from it.

This digital shrine is an exploration of my relationship to my own father and to other "father figures" in my life, both sexual and platonic. It is also a celebration of the multifaceted nature of Black and brown men, of being both hot and cold, both masculine and feminine, both sexual and intimate.

The promise of queer people coming together—across differences in region, generation, race, gender identity, and experience—has always been a utopian one. Jose Esteban Muñoz describes queer utopias as always in the distance, in the future, just out of reach. We found each other in dystopian circumstances—social unrest, global pandemics, and the rise of populist fascism domestically and abroad. Both of us have been deep in processes of creating connections between people; links to the past, present, and future; and narratives about people we know and want to know. We experience the sexualization of our queer bodies and relationships, even as we reach out to each other. Although in the queer community there are Mothers (drag mothers, gay mothers, House mothers, mothers at the job) who provide care without sexual tension, the Daddy is automatically a transaction: either for sex or money or resources.

ANDREW: Justice found me at a weird time. I was single, and my life had gotten full again with young gay and queer people of color. I have learned to be cautious and deliberate to discover what they want out of the relationship: we are often only taught to have sex with each other. He and I messaged on Instagram; we set up a call; we talked. And in that conversation, we uncovered some differences between us, as well as the same longing to be intimate. To share the space inside us with another, to touch. Justice brings passion to every conversation—asking questions, leaping down multiple paths at the same time, and wanting to know more. I respond as best I can, soothing the fire as it burns off him. We learn different ways to talk, collaborate, and commune.

JUSTICE: For years I was a flaming homosexual, catapulting through New York City with fake friends whom I believed to be my found gay family, when in actuality all we did was burn one another. I decided to make new friends, friends who could cool me down, friends to be the Obatala to my Shango.

I found Andrew in what some would say was the end of the world. I had left New York City to return home to Omaha, Nebraska, during the peak of the COVID-19 crisis. I was bummed to spend the rest of my junior year at NYU at home, but I tried to make the best of it. While writing my final paper for a "Politics of Science" course, I came across Andrew's article in the *Journal of Men's Studies* titled "Statement of Ownership: An Autoethnography of Living with HIV."

I was intrigued and inspired by Andrew's use of ethnography to humanize the experience of HIV/AIDS and how he used his experience as scientific research. So, in Generation Z fashion, I decided to direct message him on Instagram, and it has been a beautiful long-distance digital-spiritual friendship ever since. It's nice to have a friend as . . . mature as Andrew who sees your intelligence over your youth and doesn't want to fuck you. He is also a great reminder that the end of the world is just temporary and that soon I will most definitely grow into another

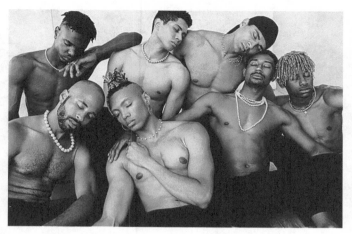
Creative Director: Justice Jamal Jones; Photography: Heather Hooton

crisis. I just have to deal with these setbacks with grace
and faith.

While being home I have also found true intimacy
with other black queers of the prairie. Dawaune Hayes
has been one of those beautiful spirits I have come across.
I cherish our friendship and spiritual intimacy. In the past
others have pushed their intentions on me as false proph-
ets, but Dawaune's real power lies in their ability to
collaborate—where the true magic is created.

Alongside Dawaune and Andrew, I have been able to
find real magic in my queerness, and I hope in our journey
that they have found the same. The visuals for this project
hope to portray that ethereal energy, with prose created
like a spell to empower other Black and brown queers to
cool down and explore their magic through intimacy.

We still have not met, not face to face. When we touch, we
know that we are calling on both this history and a vision

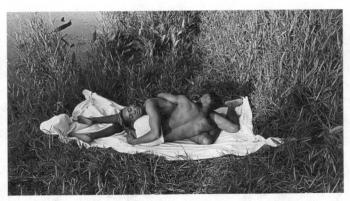

Creative Director: Justice Jamal Jones; Photography: Byron Gamble

for the future: one where two Black and Brown queers can hold each other, where cross-generational communication is not problematic or transactional. This is a divination of the world we can live in together. One lesson from the current moment: the old systems are not working, and they must be reimagined, remade, and—in some cases—abolished.

Epilogue

Promiscuity for the Non-Promiscuous

ANDREW SPIELDENNER AND
JEFFREY ESCOFFIER

Some forty years ago, psychologist Charles Silverstein launched one of the first studies of gay male couples and found that there were two strong tendencies among them that shaped gay men's relationships: some of the men tended to be "excitement seekers," whereas others tended to be "home builders." Excitement seekers emphasized novelty and change; homebuilders were more likely to stress stability and longevity. Most men were neither exclusively one or the other, and each type achieved different kinds of intimacy. The homebuilders cultivated the intimacy that develops between two people over a long period of time. But excitement seekers, who were probably more likely to be promiscuous, were also more likely to develop what sociologist Etienne Meunier calls "collective intimacy"—the kind of sexual familiarity that comes from multiple sexual encounters with people in public and in groups.[1]

One of the gay men interviewed by Silverstein summed up the situation that many gay men experienced during the 1970s:

I have a lover, but we don't put any stress on fidelity. That's not the driving force in our life, but we don't lie to each other.

Marriage is wonderful and warm and affectionate and all kinds of terrific things. One of the things it isn't is exciting, and I guess I just don't want to let go of that excitement. I've never articulated this before, but—I love the hunt. I love going out finding sex. I love cruising. I love going to the baths, cruising, prowling. . . . I'm not the most physically attractive man in the world; I'm not big and muscular. I'm twenty-five years older than most of the people, and I really like seducing and getting people to come home with me or doing it with me in the baths. I love sex itself, and I love to suck cock. I love to turn other men on because it turns me on, too.[2]

Collective intimacy is not a traditional form of personal familiarity, but it has been a historically significant form among gay men. The promiscuity and the collective intimacy that developed among gay men during the 1970s laid the foundation for the many institutions that responded to the care and support of the gay men initially infected by HIV.

Promiscuity isn't always easy for everyone involved. Like any kind of relationship, there are jerks, selfish schmucks, and emotionally naïve people. But promiscuity is important even for those who are not promiscuous—not just because it embodies an existential attitude of openness and engagement but also because the promiscuous literally create sexual opportunities.

One of the coeditors of this volume is in his late seventies and was never very promiscuous, but he has had a very pleasant sexual relationship recently with a much younger and thankfully promiscuous man. As we age, our everyday sexual perversity—which encourages all sorts of odd sexual fetishes—is an important trait of promiscuity that can often allow older men to flourish.

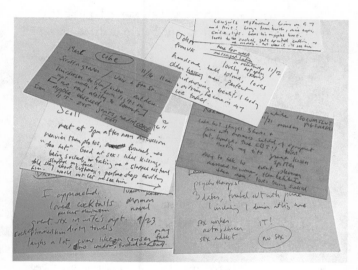

Sex cards

As Jeff Weinstein told us,

After my longtime partner died, I wanted to . . . fall in love? Hook up? That was a new phrase to me. Don, a theater critic who also became a sex therapist, told me to stop using the fussy dating sites like OK Cupid, which everyone called OK Stupid, and suggested others like Scruff (hairy) and Growlr (bears). I happened to like hair and dominant, kinky guys, and these wouldn't age-shame me, he said—I was almost 70. I also found Silver Daddies, full of youngsters, oldsters, and hetero married liars.

My doc immediately put me on Truvada, later Descovy. I worried about other STIs, but dropped that and my pants right away. I decided to keep a colored index card of each guy. Total: 32.

Random excerpts: "Paul, 40s, African, gorgeous dick, too many questions, liked to hurt my balls, not friendly, but nice message after."

"David, liked cocktails, Mormon, wrote novel, sex in wife's apartment, dirty towels, rimmed him. He came like a geyser on my mouth."

"David, from Glasgow, married, closet, sat on my face, never heard from him again. Said he had a secret boy-friend for 20 years."

"30-year-old rugby player, 250 lbs., same day as Rick, he came three times, seemed unconcerned about my pleasure."

I could go on, and I did. Until boyfriend Daniel. His card is the last.

Notes

1. Étienne Meunier, *Organizing Collective Intimacy: An Ethnography of New York City's Clandestine Sex Clubs* (New Brunswick, NJ: Rutgers University Graduate School, 2018); "Social Interaction and Safer Sex at Sex Parties: Collective and Individual Norms at Gay Group Sex Venues in NYC," *Sexuality Research and Social Policy* 15 (3): 329–341.

2. Charles Silverstein, *Man to Man: Gay Couples in America* (New York: Morrow, 1981), 114.

Acknowledgments

This book was conceived at the very moment as the Q+ Public book series. We are grateful to E. G. Crichton, the coeditor of the Q+Public book series, and the members of the Q+Public Advisory Board for their encouragement and support: Shantel Buggs, Julian Carter, Stephanie Hsu, Ajuan Mance, Maya Manvi, and Don Romesburg. We are, of course, also indebted to the contributors to this volume with whom we often had extensive discussions, who responded to our editorial suggestions with patience and grace, and who willingly revised their chapters. There are also a number of individuals who encouraged and supported each of us with critical and editorial advice—for Andrew: Roddrick Colvin, Robert Vazquez-Pacheco, José A. Romero, and the dancers at Club 69 in Puerto Vallarta who continue to inspire; and for Jeffrey: Jeffrey Colgan, Asher Horowitz, Hector Lionel, and Andrew Ragni.

Jeffrey Escoffier died suddenly after we submitted this book. *A Pill for Promiscuity* continues his work of understanding the relationships of communities and sex. Many of the contributors were friends with Jeff, and we miss him.

Notes on Contributors

PAM DORE (she/her), who is also known as Mr. Pam, is an award-winning director and cinematographer in the gay adult film industry.

JEFFREY ESCOFFIER (he/him, 1942–2022) was the coeditor of the Q+ Public series. He wrote extensively on the history of sexuality, sexual revolution, and liberation.

DANIEL FELSENTHAL (he/him) is a regular contributor to the *Village Voice* and *Pitchfork* and publishes fiction, poetry and essays, which you can read on danielfelsenthal.com.

NIC FLORES (he/him/él) is a scholar who loves cooking and tending to his plants and relationships; he wants better for himself and demands better of this world.

ALEX GARNER (he/him) is an HIV-positive, queer chicano writer and activist committed to creating change among global queer communities and currently working as the director of community engagement at MPact Global.

DEION SCOTT HAWKINS (he/him/his) is an assistant professor of Argumentation and Advocacy at Emerson College and currently serves as coalition manager for HIV Racial Justice Now!

ANDREW HOLLERAN is a novelist, essayist, and contributor to the *Gay and Lesbian Review Worldwide*.

JUSTICE JAMAL JONES describes themselves as an alchemist, combining their skills in filmmaking, writing, and acting into imaginative and passionate storytelling.

THEODORE (TED) KERR is a writer, organizer, founding member of What Would an HIV Doula Do? and coauthor of *We Are Having this Conversation Now: The Times of AIDS Cultural Production* (with Alexandra Juhasz, 2022).

LORE/TTA LEMASTER (she/they) is an artist/activist/scholar who loves donuts, tacos, and falling in love.

STEVE MACISAAC (he/him/his) is an expat Canadian living in Long Beach, California. His comics series *Shirtlifter* explores contemporary gay male culture, identity, and sexuality; see Steve's website, stevemacisaac.com.

KANE RACE is professor of Gender and Cultural Studies at the University of Sydney who works on engagement with care in the context of stigma.

ARIEL SABILLON (they/them) is a multidimensional healer and archetype integrator who works with spiritual energies to bring the body, mind, and soul into alignment with their original true essence.

ANDREW SPIELDENNER (he/him) is an advocate and academic living with HIV, who is often on the road.

ADDISON VAWTERS is a writer living in Manhattan.

Index